Cardiovascular Drugs
Vol. 4: Antihypertensive Drugs Today

Cardiovascular Drugs

Series Editor
Graeme S. Avery, Auckland

Editor-in-Chief
Australasian Drug Information Services
Sydney · Auckland
Editor
Drugs · Clinical Pharmacokinetics

MTPPRESS LIMITED *International Medical Publishers*

Antihypertensive Drugs Today
Vol. 4 in Cardiovascular Drugs

With 14 figures and 18 tables

MTPPRESS LIMITED *International Medical Publishers*

Antihypertensive Drugs Today
Vol. 4 in Cardiovascular Drugs

Published in UK, Europe and Middle East
by MTP Press Limited
Falcon House
Lancaster
England

Companion volumes

Cardiovascular Drugs Vol. 1: Antiarrhythmic, Antihypertensive
and Lipid Lowering Drugs ISBN 0-9599827-6-0
Cardiovascular Drugs Vol. 2: β-Adrenoceptor Blocking Drugs
ISBN-13: 978-94-011-7270-7   e-ISBN-13: 978-94-011-7268-4
DOI: 10.1007/978-94-011-7268-4
Cardiovascular Drugs Vol. 3: Antithrombotic Drugs
ISBN-13: 978-94-011-7270-7

Cardiovascular Drugs Vol. 4

ISBN-13: 978-94-011-7270-7

First Printing

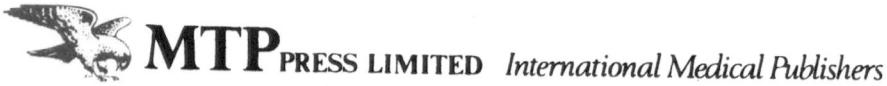

MTPPRESS LIMITED *International Medical Publishers*

Editor's Note

As with the previous volumes in the *Cardiovascular Drugs* series, *Antihypertensive Drugs Today* is designed to provide undergraduate and postgraduate students, and physicians in practice, with a state of the art review of the pharmacological properties and therapeutic use of a group of drugs.

In the first section of the book Professor Wollam and his colleagues deal with the whole range of antihypertensive drugs, ending their review with an exposition of the 'stepped care' programme which enables a rational choice of the various agents, taking into account the degree of hypertension and its response to previous therapy. The rest of the volume is devoted to a more detailed account of three of the more recently introduced drugs of importance in hypertension: the cardioselective β-adrenoceptor blocker, metoprolol; the α- and β-adrenoceptor blocking agent, labetalol and, finally, prazosin, which owes its antihypertensive activity to peripheral vasodilation consequent to post-synaptic α-adrenoceptor blockade.

Each chapter in this book has previously appeared as a review article in the ADIS Press journal, *Drugs:* the authors have revised and up-dated them for this volume. The manuscripts for the articles on metoprolol, labetalol and prazosin were each reviewed by a panel of international experts (see Acknowledgements) and my colleagues and I would like to record our thanks to all of them for their advice and encouragement.

14 June 1979   R.N. Brogden

Contributors

Avery, G.S.
Australasian Drug Information Services, Auckland, New Zealand.

Brogden, R.N.
Australasian Drug Information Services, Auckland, New Zealand.

Gifford, R.W., Jr.
Department of Hypertension and Nephrology, Cleveland Clinic Foundation, Cleveland, Ohio, USA.

Heel, R.C.
Australasian Drug Information Services, Auckland, New Zealand.

Speight, T.M.
Australasian Drug Information Services, Auckland, New Zealand.

Tarazi, R.C.
Clinical Section, Research Division, Cleveland Clinic Foundation, Cleveland, Ohio, USA.

Wollam, G.L.
Division of Hypertension, Emory University School of Medicine, Atlanta, Georgia, USA.

Contents of Volume 4

Chapter I

Antihypertensive Drugs: Clinical Pharmacology and Therapeutic Use 1

G.L. Wollam, R.W. Gifford, Jr. and R.C. Tarazi

Chapter II

Metoprolol: A Review of its Pharmacological Properties and Therapeutic Efficacy in Hypertension

R.N. Brogden, R.C. Heel, T.M. Speight and G.S. Avery

Chapter III

Labetalol: A Review of its Pharmacology and Therapeutic Use in Hypertension 100

R.N. Brogden, R.C. Heel, T.M. Speight and G.S. Avery

Chapter IV

Prazosin: A Review of its Pharmacological Properties and Therapeutic Efficacy in Hypertension 125

R.N. Brogden, R.C. Heel, T.M. Speight and G.S. Avery

Contents of Volume 1
Antiarrhythmic, Antihypertensive and Lipid Lowering Drugs

Contents

Chapter III

Antiarrhythmic Agents: Mechanisms of Action, Clinical Pharmacology and Therapeutic Considerations

D.T. Mason, A.N. DeMaria, E.A. Amsterdam, L.A. Vismara, R.R. Miller, Z. Vera, G. Lee, R. Zelis and R.A. Massumi

Chapter IV

Clinical Pharmacology and Therapeutic Use of Digitalis Glycosides

J.E. Doherty and J.J. Kane

Contents of Volume 2
β-Adrenoceptor Blocking Drugs

Chapter IV

β-Adrenoreceptor Blocking Drugs in Angina Pectoris

B.N.C. Prichard

Chapter V

β-Adrenoreceptor Blocking Drugs in Cardiac Arrhythmias

B.N. Singh and D.E. Jewitt

Chapter VI

β-Adrenoreceptor Blocking Drugs in Hyperthyroidism

D.G. McDevitt and R.G. Shanks

Chapter VII

Clinical Toxicity of Propranolol and Practolol: A Report from the Boston Collaborative Drug Surveillance Program

D.J. Greenblatt and J. Koch-Weser

Chapter VIII

Adverse Effects of β-Adrenoreceptor Blocking Drugs on Respiration

H.M. Beumer

Chapter IX

Autoimmune Phenomena and Autoallergy in Patients Treated with β-Adrenoreceptor Blocking Drugs

E.S.K. Assem

Contents of Volume 3
Antithrombotic Drugs

Chapter I

Platelets, Thrombosis and Drugs

J.F. Mustard and Marian A. Packham

Chapter I

Antihypertensive Drugs:
Clinical Pharmacology and Therapeutic Use

G.L. Wollam, R.W. Gifford, Jr. and R.C. Tarazi

Knowledge of clinical pharmacology is an important prerequisite to the rational use of drugs. This is especially true of antihypertensive therapy because the ever increasing number of antihypertensive agents allows the clinician wide latitude in his selection of a suitable regimen. An understanding of the clinical pharmacology of antihypertensive drugs allows a more rational approach to therapy and permits a finer tuning of individual drug regimens.

There is an ever increasing number of antihypertensive agents available to clinicians. They may be classified according to their primary mode of action (table I).

1. Diuretics

The diuretics have been shown to reduce blood pressure regardless of their chemical composition or site of action on the renal tubule, and when administered in equivalent pharmacological dosages, they have a similar antihypertensive effect (Dustan et al., 1974). Approximately 30 % of patients with mild to moderate hypertension will achieve adequate blood pressure control with a diuretic alone. Because of this high success rate and the low incidence of side effects, diuretic therapy is widely recommended as the initial treatment for mild to moderate hypertension.

1.1 Mechanism of Action

Although the exact means by which diuretics lower blood pressure is not completely understood, the physiological events which occur with diuretic treatment have

Table I. Classification of antihypertensive agents

1. *Diuretics*
    a) 'Thiazide' type.
    b) 'Loop' diuretics — frusemide, ethacrynic acid.
    c) Potassium sparing agents — spironolactone, amiloride, triamterene.

2. *Sympathetic inhibitors*
    a) Central action — clonidine.
    b) Ganglion blocking agents — trimetaphan, pentolinium, pempidine.
    c) Blockade of neuroeffector transmission — guanethidine, bethanidine, debrisoquine; reserpine.
    d) Combined central and peripheral action — methyldopa.
    e) Adrenoceptor blocking agents.
        i) α-Adrenoceptor blockade — phentolamine, phenoxybenzamine (pre- and post-synaptic blockade); prazosin (post-synaptic blockade).
        ii) β-Adrenoceptor blockade — non-selective (combined β_1 and β_2 blockade); cardioselective (predominantly β_1 blockade) [see also table III].
        iii) Combined α- and β-adrenoceptor blockade — labetalol.
    f) Undefined action — MAO inhibitors (pargyline).

3. *Direct acting vasodilators*
    a) Arterial — hydrallazine, diazoxide, minoxidil.
    b) Arterial and venous — sodium nitroprusside.

4. *Angiotensin II analogues and converting enzyme inhibitors* — saralasin; compound SQ20881

been fairly well elucidated. The immediate effect is a reduction in plasma and extracellular fluid volume which is accompanied by a fall in cardiac output. The total peripheral resistance is increased in the early stage of therapy and initially, the reduction in arterial pressure is brought about by a decrease in cardiac output (Dustan et al., 1974; Dustan et al., 1959; Frohlich et al., 1960). After a period of several weeks, long term haemodynamic adjustments occur; the cardiac output returns to pretreatment levels as total peripheral resistance falls. The exact nature of these systemic readjustments is not well understood.

It has been shown that diuretics reduce vascular resistance (Conway and Palmero, 1963; Ogilvie and Schlieper, 1970), and the pressor responses to infusions of noradrenaline (Freis et al., 1960; Mendlowitz et al., 1960; Frohlich et al., 1972; Feisal et al., 1961) and angiotensin II (Abboud, 1974; Heistad et al., 1971). Possibly, diuretic induced sodium depletion interferes with the ability of the sympathetic nervous system to adapt to changes in intravascular volume, or it may be a response of the peripheral vasculature to the reduction in cardiac output (so-called autoregulation).

In the final analysis, the reduction in blood pressure with long term therapy is maintained by a diminished total peripheral resistance (Tarazi, 1973a; Lund-

Johansen, 1970; Conway and Lauwers, 1960), associated with a persistent reduction in plasma and extracellular fluid volume (Leth, 1970; Tarazi and Dustan, 1977; Tarazi et al., 1970). The extracellular fluid contraction may not be as marked as in the initial stages, possibly because of increased proximal reabsorption of sodium and secondary aldosteronism. Thus, throughout diuretic therapy, arterial pressure is reduced through the interplay of two mechanisms: a contraction of the extracellular fluid and plasma volume and an inadequate cardiovascular compensation for the degree of hypovolaemia.

1.2 Pharmacokinetics

1.2.1 Thiazide-like Diuretics
The benzothiadiazine ('thiazide') diuretics and closely related analogues such as chlorthalidone and metolazone are, in general, well absorbed from the gastrointestinal tract (Mudge, 1975). About 30 to 60 % of orally administered chlorothiazide is systemically absorbed (Brettell et al., 1960; Baer et al., 1959), whereas 60 to 80 % of orally administered hydrochlorothiazide is absorbed following oral administration (Anderson et al., 1961; Beermann et al., 1976). Absorption from the gastrointestinal tract is almost complete for some of the more highly substituted benzothiadazine derivatives such as bendroflumethiazide (Brettell et al., 1964) and polythiazide (Pinson et al., 1962).

The onset of diuresis usually occurs within 1 to 2 hours following oral administration with most agents (Mudge, 1975); however, the various thiazide diuretics differ considerably with regard to their duration of action. The shorter acting drugs such as chlorothiazide, hydrochlorothiazide, benzthiazide and hydroflumethiazide have their major natriuretic effect within 4 to 8 hours following oral administration and their diuretic action subsides within 12 to 18 hours (Murphy et al., 1961; Ford and Bush, 1960; Fuchs et al., 1960; Davies and Wilson, 1975; Kennedy et al., 1959). The longer acting thiazide diuretics such as methyclothiazide (Ford and Bush, 1960), trichlormethiazide (Taylor and Maren, 1963), cyclothiazide (Swartz et al., 1963), bendroflumethiazide (Piala et al., 1961) and polythiazide (Ford, 1961) are effective for up to 24 hours or longer. In the case of polythiazide and the phthalimidine derivative chlorthalidone, the natriuretic effect may persist for as long as 72 hours (Hutcheon and Leonard, 1963; Mees and Geyskes, 1964).

Variations in the duration of action among the thiazide diuretics does not appear to be closely related to differences in gastrointestinal absorption or metabolic transformation (Davies and Wilson, 1975; Peters and Roch-Ramel, 1969) but seem best correlated with the rate of elimination of the various drugs, which is largely determined by certain physiochemical characteristics such as binding to plasma proteins, volume of distribution and lipid solubility (Peters and Roch-Ramel, 1969; Lant and Wilson, 1972; Beyer and Baer, 1975).

The shorter acting drugs, such as chlorothiazide, are less bound to plasma proteins and exhibit relatively poor lipid solubility. Consequently they are largely confined to the extracellular water and are rapidly excreted by the kidney (Davies and Wilson, 1975; Peters and Roch-Ramel, 1969; Lant and Wilson, 1972).

By contrast, the longer acting thiazides are more highly protein bound, exhibit greater lipid solubility and have a larger volume of distribution within the body (Davies and Wilson, 1975; Peters and Roch-Ramel, 1969; Lant and Wilson, 1972; Beyer and Baer, 1975). The longer duration of action of these agents seems roughly correlated with their slower rate of elimination and greater liposolubility, which presumably allows greater cellular penetration and binding to tissue storage sites '(Davies and Wilson, 1975; Beyer and Baer, 1975). Furthermore, the greater protein binding of the longer acting drugs reduces their renal clearance and prolongs their diuretic action (Davies and Wilson, 1975). There is some evidence to suggest that their increased liposolubility permits passive back diffusion to occur in the distal nephron which may further diminish urinary excretion (Beyer and Baer, 1975; Scriabine et al., 1962; Duggan, 1966; Peters and Roch-Ramel, 1969); however, this remains controversial.

Renal excretion constitutes the major route of elimination of the thiazide diuretics and is accomplished by both glomerular filtration and tubular secretion (Beyer and Baer, 1975). Most of these agents are excreted in the urine unchanged (Davies and Wilson, 1975); however, some of the longer acting derivatives such as bendroflumethiazide, trichlormethiazide and polythiazide may be partially metabolised (Pinson et al., 1962; Peters and Roch-Ramel, 1969). The thiazide diuretics are excreted in the bile in small amounts and there is some evidence to suggest that a limited degree of enterohepatic circulation may occur (Peters and Roch-Ramel, 1969; Baer et al., 1959; Hart and Schanker, 1966; Sheppard et al., 1960; Beyer, 1958). Although the data are incomplete, current evidence would suggest that less than 5% of chlorothiazide and hydrochlorothiazide is excreted by the biliary tree in patients with normal renal function (Calesnick et al., 1961). However, animal studies suggest that a much larger portion may be eliminated by biliary secretion in renal insufficiency (Baer et al., 1959). Excretion of the thiazide diuretics is prolonged in patients with renal insufficiency (Brettell et al., 1960; Anderson et al., 1961; Beerman et al., 1976; Brettell et al., 1964). Urinary excretion and possibly gastrointestinal absorption may be impaired in some patients with cardiac and hepatic decompensation (Brettell et al., 1960; Anderson et al., 1961; Brettell et al., 1964).

Chlorthalidone and metolazone are sulphonamide diuretics which differ chemically from the thiazide diuretics in that a phthalimidine group, in chlorthalidone, and a quinazoline group, in metolazone, has been substituted into the benzothiadiazine heterocyclic ring structure (Mudge, 1975). Pharmacologically, however, the mode of action of these agents is identical to the thiazide diuretics (Suki et al., 1965, 1972).

Chlorthalidone is slowly, but almost completely absorbed following oral administration and peak blood levels are achieved within 6 to 8 hours (Pulver et al., 1959; Tweeddale and Ogilvie, 1974). It appears to be widely distributed throughout the body, with the exception of adipose tissue and lipid-rich organs such as the central nervous system, and it is heavily concentrated in the kidney (Pulver et al., 1959) and erythrocytes (Beerman et al., 1975). There is preferential and prolonged binding to renal tissue (Pulver et al., 1959) which together with the slow absorption and relative freedom from metabolic degradation, probably accounts for its prolonged duration of action (Mees and Geyskes, 1964). Only 30 to 60% of an orally administered dose is excreted unchanged in the urine (Tweeddale and Ogilvie, 1974) and animal studies have suggested that some biliary excretion with enterohepatic circulation may occur (Beisenherz et al., 1966).

Metolazone appears to be readily absorbed by the gastrointestinal tract (Hinsvark and Cohen, 1970). The onset of diuresis begins within 2 hours (Steinmuller and Puschett, 1972) and may persist for 18 hours or more (Goldberg et al., 1977). Metolazone is highly bound by plasma proteins, is taken up by erythrocytes and has a large volume of distribution (Costa et al., unpublished observations). It appears to undergo partial metabolic degradation and is excreted by the kidney and to a lesser extent by the biliary system (Costa et al., unpublished observations; Cohen et al., 1973).

1.2.2 'Loop' Diuretics

Ethacrynic acid is a derivative of phenoxyacetic acid, whereas frusemide is a sulphanylbenzene derivative of anthranilic acid and is structurally related to the benzothiadiazine diuretics (Goldberg, 1973).

Frusemide is rapidly absorbed following oral administration and gastrointestinal absorption accounts for approximately 40 to 76% of the administered dose (Rupp, 1974; Kelly et al., 1974; Huang et al., 1974; Calesnick et al., 1966). When ingested in the fasting state, serum levels are detectable within 10 minutes and peak serum concentrations are achieved within 60 to 70 minutes. Following postprandial administration, absorption is delayed in comparison with fasting administration; however, total drug absorption and the net diuretic effect are not significantly different (Kelly et al., 1974).

The onset of diuresis occurs within 20 to 60 minutes following oral administration. The peak natriuresis occurs at 2 hours and the diuresis terminates within 6 to 8 hours (Kim et al., 1971). With intravenous administration, the onset of diuresis is extremely rapid (within 5 minutes). The maximal effect is observed within 30 minutes and diuresis is usually completed within 2 hours (Kelly et al., 1974; Goldberg, 1973). With both frusemide and ethacrynic acid, the maximum diuresis following intravenous administration can be quite striking, and peak urine flow rates as high as 30ml/min (approaching 20 to 30% of glomerular filtration) have been reported (Robson et al., 1964).

Frusemide is highly bound to plasma proteins (95 %) and does not appear to undergo extensive metabolic transformation (Kelly et al., 1974). In the presence of normal renal function frusemide is rapidly excreted by the kidney, both by glomerular filtration and tubular secretion (Calesnick et al., 1966; Cutler et al., 1974). Following intravenous administration, 80 to 92 % appears in the urine within 24 hours, most of which (about 77 %) is excreted within 4 hours, and the plasma half-life is approximately 30 minutes (Calesnick et al., 1966; Cutler et al., 1974). The remaining 8 to 12 % is eliminated by non-renal mechanisms, presumably by biliary excretion (Rupp, 1974; Beermann et al., 1977). In chronic renal insufficiency, the plasma half-life is markedly prolonged (3 to 20 hours) [Huang et al., 1974]. Urinary excretion of frusemide is reduced in proportion to glomerular filtration (Rose et al., 1977) and a correspondingly greater amount is eliminated by non-renal mechanisms presumably in the bile (Rupp, 1974; Huang et al., 1974; Cutler et al., 1974). In uraemic patients, up to 98 % of the administered dose is eliminated within 24 hours by non-renal mechanisms, and accumulation is effectively prevented in the absence of hepatic dysfunction (Huang et al., 1974). Possibly because gastrointestinal absorption appears to be erratic in some patients with advanced renal insufficiency, intravenous administration is often more effective in eliciting a diuretic response (Huang et al., 1974; Greither et al., 1976).

The pharmacokinetics of ethacrynic acid are not well understood. However, like frusemide, ethacrynic acid appears to be rapidly absorbed from the gastrointestinal tract (Davies and Wilson, 1975). With either oral or intravenous administration, the onset and duration of action, as well as the diuretic potency of ethacrynic acid is similar to that of frusemide (Kim et al., 1971).

Ethacrynic acid is highly bound to plasma proteins (Davies and Wilson, 1975) and undergoes rapid elimination by the kidney and biliary system (Lant and Wilson, 1972). Approximately one-third is excreted in the bile and two-thirds in the urine in the form of unchanged ethacrynic acid, a cysteine adduct or unidentified metabolites (Mudge, 1975; Beyer et al., 1965). There is evidence to suggest that the mode of action may involve the formation of an ethacrynic-cysteine complex, which acts within the lumen of the nephron to inhibit active chloride reabsorption in the region of the thick medullary portion of the ascending limb of the loop of Henle (Burg and Green, 1973).

1.2.3 Potassium-sparing Agents (spironolactone, triamterene, amiloride)

Spironolactone is readily absorbed following oral administration and bioavailability is estimated at 60 to 70 % (Sadee et al., 1973; Karim et al., 1976a). Following absorption, spironolactone is rapidly and almost completely metabolised to canrenone (about 80 %) and several other metabolites including 6-betahydroxysulphoxide and canrenoate (Karim et al., 1976a; Karim et al., 1976b; Sadee et al., 1973). Canrenone is probably the principal pharmacologically active agent responsible for the anti-mineralocorticoid effect of spironolactone (Davies and Wilson, 1975; Ramsay et al., 1977). Peak serum levels of canrenone appear within 3 hours following ingestion of spironolactone (Karim et al., 1976a). Canrenone is highly protein bound (90%) and elimination occurs with a rapid decline in serum levels over 12 hours (half-life 4 hours) followed by a slower rate of decline over 72 hours (half-life 17 hours) [Karim et al., 1976a]. The slow rate of elimination of canrenone suggests that twice daily administration may be sufficient in many patients (Karim et al., 1976c). Canrenone and the other metabolites of spironolactone are largely excreted in the urine (Karim et al., 1976a); however, animal studies have indicated that biliary excretion may also occur (Sadee et al., 1974).

Triamterene is rapidly absorbed from the gasrointestinal tract; however, absorption is extremely variable among individuals ranging from 30 to 70% (Pruitt et al., 1977). Peak plasma concentrations are observed within 2 to 4 hours and the plasma half-life is 90 to 120 minutes in normal subjects (Pruitt et al., 1977). The maximal pharmacological effect is observed at approximately 2 to 4 hours and terminates within 10 hours (Davies and Wilson, 1975; Baba et al., 1962). Triamterene undergoes rapid and extensive metabolic transformation, presumably in the liver, to form a p-hydroxyphenyl metabolite. Because of the rapid rate of biotransformation, the plasma concentration of this metabolite may increase to as much as 12 times that of unconverted triamterene. The metabolic conversion to the p-hydroxyphenyl metabolite appears to be significantly reduced in the presence of hepatic dysfunction. Preliminary studies of this metabolite in animals have failed to reveal any evidence of diuretic activity; however, studies in man are lacking (Pruitt et al., 1977). Triamterene is partially bound to plasma proteins (43 to 54%) and, together with the p-hydroxyphenyl metabolite, is rapidly excreted by the kidney, most of which appears in the urine within 24 hours (Pruitt et al., 1977; Lassen and Nielsen, 1963); however small amounts are also eliminated by biliary secretion.

Amiloride is moderately well absorbed (20 to 50% from the gastrointestinal tract) [Weiss et al., 1969]. Maximal serum concentrations are achieved within 3 to 4 hours and decline with a half-life of approximately 6 hours (Weiss et al., 1969). The onset of action occurs approximately 2 hours following oral administration. The maximal pharmacological effect is achieved at 6 to 10 hours and persists for up to 24 hours (Davies and Wilson, 1975). Amiloride does not undergo significant biotransformation and is excreted by the kidney, most appearing in the urine within 48 hours (Weiss et al., 1969; Grayson et al., 1971).

1.3 Clinical Use

Although the various classes of diuretics (table II) behave similarly in regard to their antihypertensive effect, there are certain indications for choosing a given diuretic agent.

Table II. Classification and dosages of oral diuretics used in the management of hypertension

Diuretic	Dosage		
	Minimal	Usual	Maximal
1. *Sulphonamide derivatives*			
a) Benzothiadiazine compounds			
Chlorothiazide	500mg qd	500mg bid	500mg tid
Hydrochlorothiazide	50mg qd	50mg bid	50mg tid
Bendroflazide	5mg qd	10mg qd	15mg qd
Methychlothiazide	5mg qd	10mg qd	15mg qd
Hydroflumethiazide	50mg qd	50mg bid	50mg tid
Benzthiazide	50mg qd	50mg bid	50mg tid
Polythiazide	2mg qd	4mg qd	8mg qd
Cyclothiazide	2mg qd	4mg qd	6mg qd
Trichlormethiazide	2mg qd	4mg qd	8mg qd
b) Phthalimidine compound			
Chlorthalidone	50mg qd	50mg qd	100mg qd
c) Quinazoline compounds			
Quinethazone	50mg qd	50mg bid	50mg tid
Metolazone	2.5mg qd	5.0mg qd	10mg qd
d) Anthranilic acid compound			
Frusemide (furosemide)[1]	40mg bid	40mg qid	500mg bid or more
2. *Phenoxyacetic acid derivative*			
Ethacrynic acid[1]	50mg bid	50mg qid	500mg bid or more
3. *Distal tubular diuretics*			
Spironolactone	25mg bid	25mg qid	100mg qid
Amiloride	5mg qd	5mg bid	10mg bid
Triamterene	100mg qd	100mg bid	100mg tid

1 'Loop' diuretics have a steep dose response curve and are effective when renal function is impaired whereas the others are not.

1.3.1 Thiazide-like Diuretics

The benzothiadiazine ('thiazide') diuretics and closely related drugs such as chlorthalidone and metolazone, have the widest scope of usefulness in the treatment of hypertension. They are all quite similar in regard to their pharmacological effects, and there is very little therapeutic advantage in the choice of one particular agent over another. They differ mainly in their duration of action and the shorter acting preparations need to be administered twice daily to achieve maximum therapeutic benefit.

The thiazide-like diuretics act by interfering with sodium and chloride reabsorption in the distal cortical diluting segment of the renal tubule, where approximately 5 % of sodium reabsorption occurs. All drugs in this group may cause hypokalaemia, hyperuricaemia and hyperglycaemia (Shapiro et al., 1961; Goldner et al., 1960). The thiazides decrease calcium excretion and on rare occasions produce hypercalcaemia. The presence of persistent hypercalcaemia in a patient being treated with a thiazide diuretic may be indicative of an underlying parathyroid adenoma (Duarte et al., 1971).

1.3.2 'Loop' Diuretics

The so-called 'loop' diuretics, frusemide (furosemide) and ethacrynic acid, have their major action on the ascending limb of the loop of Henle where about 20 % of the reabsorption of sodium and chloride occurs. They are the most potent of the available diuretic agents. As they have a relatively short duration of action, however, they must be administered 3 or 4 times daily to obtain an antihypertensive effect equivalent to that of the thiazides (Anderson et al., 1971).

Because of the frequency of administration and the rapid onset of diuresis, which is disturbing to many patients, the loop diuretics are somewhat less convenient than the thiazide diuretics. However, they have a distinct advantage in patients with renal insufficiency because they have a steep dose response curve and large doses are effective even when glomerular filtration is severely impaired (Reubi, 1966). In contrast, the thiazide and related diuretics have a flat dose response curve (maximum effective dose for chlorothiazide is 1,500mg and for hydrochlorothiazide 150mg) and, because of their lesser potency, are ineffective in severe renal insufficiency (Reubi and Cottier, 1961). Moreover, the thiazide diuretics may reduce glomerular filtration rate and aggravate azotaemia (Villarreal et al., 1962), whereas the loop diuretics maintain the glomerular filtration rate and may actually increase it (Reubi, 1966).

Frusemide is preferable to ethacrynic acid in patients with severe renal insufficiency because the latter is associated with a higher incidence of gastrointestinal side effects, including nausea, vomiting, diarrhoea and abdominal distention. The combination of a thiazide diuretic and frusemide is often effective in patients with azotaemia who have responded inadequately to treatment with frusemide alone (Wollam et al., 1977).

1.3.3 Potassium-sparing Agents (spironolactone, amiloride, triamterene)

Spironolactone is a mild diuretic agent which acts on the mineralocorticoid portion of the distal tubule to inhibit the aldosterone dependent sodium-for-potassium exchange. It is occasionally used to reverse or prevent diuretic induced hypokalaemia in patients who are taking digitalis and in the treatment of primary aldosteronism. It should be used in relatively small doses, 25 to 50mg four times a day to minimise or avoid oestrogen-like side effects, and should be combined with a thiazide diuretic to enhance the diuretic effect. It must be employed with caution in patients with diminished renal function as it has the potential for causing hyperkalaemia.

Spironolactone does not cause hyperglycaemia or hypercalcaemia and rarely produces hyperuricaemia; however, because of its steroidal activity, it may cause gynaecomastia, impotence and menometrorrhagia. It should be remembered that aspirin, in modest doses, can completely inhibit the effect of spironolactone on the distal tubule (Tweeddale and Ogilvie, 1973).

Amiloride and triamterene, like spironolactone, are mild diuretic agents which act on the distal convoluted tubule. However, the ability of these drugs to diminish urinary potassium excretion is achieved by a direct action on the sodium-for-potassium exchange mechanism rather than by competitive antagonism of aldosterone. As with spironolactone, they are used to reverse or prevent diuretic-induced hypokalaemia. Side effects are fewer than with spironolactone; hyperkalaemia represents the most serious side effect and this can occur when the drugs are used in combination with thiazide diuretics (Davies and Wilson, 1975).

1.4 Side Effects

Asymptomatic diuretic induced hypokalaemia is harmless unless the patient has myocardial disease and/or is taking digitalis, in which case serious arrhythmias can occur. The most effective and reliable way to prevent diuretic induced hypokalaemia when it is advisable to do so is to add a potassium-sparing agent such as spironolactone to the regimen.

Asymptomatic diuretic induced hyperuricaemia is also usually harmless. If the patient has a history of gout or develops gout, the diuretic should be continued and the gout should be treated with probenecid or allopurinol, plus colchicine. Diuretic induced hyperglycaemia is usually clinically insignificant. Occasionally in diabetic patients, however, the addition of a thiazide type of diuretic to the regimen will require closer dietary management and/or adjustment in the dosage of the hypoglycaemic agent(s). Diabetes and gout are not contraindications to the use of thiazide or loop diuretics.

Photosensitivity is a rare side effect of the sulphonamide diuretics (Harber et al., 1959) but has not been reported with ethacrynic acid or the potassium-sparing drugs.

Ototoxicity with hearing loss has been infrequently associated with the administration of ethacrynic acid and is usually reversible but is occasionally permanent (Mathog and Klein, 1969; Cooperman and Rubin, 1973; Mathog et al., 1970). Transient hearing loss has been reported with frusemide (Schwartz et al., 1970; Wigand and Heidland, 1971). The hearing loss can be associated with tinnitus or vertigo and most often occurs following the parenteral administration of large doses of ethacrynic acid or frusemide to patients with renal insufficiency. Allergic interstitial nephritis with renal failure, which is often reversible, is also a rare side effect of the thiazide diuretics and frusemide (Lyons et al., 1973).

2. Sympathetic Inhibiting Agents

2.1 Ganglionic Blocking Agents

The significance of the ganglionic blocking drugs is probably of more historical than practical importance. With the availability of sodium nitroprusside and drugs which selectively inhibit the adrenergic nervous system, these agents are seldom, if ever, used. However, intravenous preparations (e.g. triametaphan camsylate) are occasionally used for the treatment of hypertensive emergencies.

These compounds act on the autonomic ganglia by preventing the attachment of the neurotransmitter, acetylcholine, to the receptor sites of the postganglionic axon (Volle and Koelle, 1975). They block the transmission of both sympathetic and parasympathetic impulses and are among the most potent antihypertensive drugs available. The fall in blood pressure is mediated by a reduction in cardiac output, which is due to pooling of blood in venous capacitance vessels (Aviado, 1960), without a direct depressant effect on the myocardium (Lee and Shideman, 1958). The peripheral resistance may also be reduced in the acute treatment phase (Bhatia and Frohlich, 1973; Tarazi and Dustan, 1973).

Marked orthostatic hypotension is a characteristic feature of ganglionic blocking agents and this can be utilised therapeutically by tilting the head of the bed or by the addition of diuretic therapy. The associated parasympathetic blockade produces severe and disabling side effects including blurred vision, dryness of the mouth, constipation, paralytic ileus, urinary retention and impotence. For this reason, the ganglionic blocking agents have been superseded by newer agents which selectively inhibit the sympathetic nervous system.

2.2 Guanethidine and Other Adrenergic Neurone Blocking Drugs

Guanethidine is a powerful antihypertensive agent with a potency similar to the ganglionic blockers. Since its introduction over 15 years ago, guanethidine has proved to be an extremely effective antihypertensive agent and has been widely used in the treatment of moderate to severe hypertension. However, with the addition of newer sympatholytic agents with fewer annoying untoward effects, it is now generally reserved for the treatment of severe hypertension which is resistant to other agents.

2.2.1 Mechanism of Action

Guanethidine is a selective inhibitor of the sympathetic nervous system and does not interfere with parasympathetic function (Freis, 1965). It acts at the level of the postganglionic adrenergic neurone by inhibiting the release of noradrenaline at the neuroeffector junction, which occurs in response to sympathetic stimulation (Hertting et al., 1962). In order to be effective, guanethidine and the other guanidinium compounds such as bethanidine and debrisoquine, must be actively transported into the adrenergic neurone by the 'noradrenaline pump' (Mitchell and Oates, 1970). Once it gains access to the neurone, guanethidine accumulates within the intraneuronal storage vesicles and causes depletion of noradrenaline stores within the nerve terminal (Chang et al., 1965). Although it is released from storage vesicles with noradrenaline in response to sympathetic nerve stimulation, it does not act as a false transmitter and its sympatholytic action does not depend directly upon the level of noradrenaline depletion (Shand et al., 1973; Gaffney et al., 1963). In fact, the exact mode of action has not been completely clarified. There is some evidence to indicate, however, that possibly the major mode of action may reside in the inhibition of nerve pulse transmission at the level of the outer neuronal or vesicular membranes within the sympathetic nerve terminal (Shand et al., 1973).

The intravenous administration of guanethidine produces a transient pressor response with increased cardiac output and peripheral vasoconstriction (Cohn et al., 1963; Page et al., 1961) due in part to the liberation of catecholamines from adrenergic nerve terminals (Harrison et al., 1963). The pressor response generally lasts for less than an hour and is followed by a reduction in arterial pressure as the terminal sympathetic neurones become unresponsive to electrical stimulation (Freis, 1965). Tissue catecholamines are not reduced during the early treatment phase; however, with chronic treatment, catecholamine stores are slowly depleted, probably as the result of impaired storage mechanisms (Harrison et al., 1963).

The prolonged oral administration of guanethidine produces a 'denervation sensitivity' of the neuroeffector junction (Abboud et al., 1962). This probably results from the chronic reduction in the amount of noradrenaline released by the sympathetic nerve endings. Systemic responses to catecholamines released from the adrenal medulla are not prevented and may even be augmented as a result of this denervation sensitivity (Boura and Green, 1965; Richardson and Wyso, 1960). Thus, a paradoxical hypertensive crisis may occur if guanethidine is administered to patients with phaeochromocytoma, or if noradrenaline is given to a patient receiving the drug.

Because of poor lipid solubility guanethidine does not cross the blood-brain barrier and is not associated with central nervous system side effects which are so prominent with other sympatholytic agents such as reserpine, clonidine and methyldopa. In contrast to most neural blocking agents, guanethidine does not appear to suppress plasma renin activity in many patients (Ferguson et al., 1976). In fact, in some patients with essential hypertension and suppressed plasma renin activity, guanethidine has been observed to stimulate renin secretion to the range of 'normal renin hypertension' (Lowder and Liddle, 1975). This remains controversial, however.

The haemodynamic changes which occur with guanethidine in the early phase of treatment are characterised by a fall in cardiac output and little or no change in peripheral vascular resistance (Cohn et al., 1963; Richardson et al., 1960; Onesti et al., 1973). The reduction in arterial pressure is greater in the upright position as a result of a further reduction in cardiac output due to gravitational pooling of blood in the lower extremities, and failure of a compensatory rise in peripheral resistance (Richardson et al., 1960; Richardson and Wyso, 1960). With long term therapy, haemodynamic adjustments occur and the cardiac output gradually increases to near pretreatment levels while the peripheral resistance gradually falls (Chamberlain and Howard, 1964; Villarreal et al., 1964). A significant reduction in both renal blood flow and glomerular filtration rate occurs in the acute treatment phase (Richardson et al., 1960; Onesti et al., 1973). Although there are no studies of the long term effects on renal haemodynamics, chronic therapy is not generally associated with clinically significant changes in renal function (Page et al., 1961; Woosley and Nies, 1976).

2.2.2 Pharmacokinetics
Systemic absorption of orally administered guanethidine is extremely variable among individuals and ranges between 3 and 27% of the administered dose (McMartin and Simpson, 1971). However, for a given patient, gastrointestinal absorption appears to be relatively constant (McMartin and Simpson, 1971). Once the oral dose reaches the systemic circulation, it is rapidly distributed to tissue storage sites, including adrenergic neurones (McMartin et al., 1970).

Guanethidine has a serum half-life of about 5 days (Shand et al., 1975). With chronic therapy, it is estimated that about 1/7 of the total body pool is eliminated each day (Shand et al., 1975) and approximately three half-lives (about 15 days) are required to achieve steady state levels (Woosley and Nies, 1976). Guanethidine is excreted almost entirely by the kidney (McMartin and Simpson, 1971).

2.2.3 Clinical Use
Guanethidine and the related drugs bethanidine and debrisoquine are among the most potent antihypertensive agents currently available for oral administration. Because they frequently produce annoying side effects, they are generally reserved for treatment of severe hypertension, which is resistant to other antihypertensive agents.

The sympathoplegic action of guanethidine leads to expansion of the intravascular volume which produces tolerance to its antihypertensive effect (Freis, 1965; Smith, 1965a; Dustan et al., 1972). The plasma volume expansion results from a shift of interstitial fluid into the intravascular compartment in the early phase of treatment (Weil and Chidsey, 1968), and sodium and fluid retention with long term therapy (Smith, 1965b). Therefore, guanethidine should always be used in combination with a diuretic agent. It is often advisable to include methyldopa in the antihypertensive regimen also as the dosage requirement for guanethidine is generally reduced, thereby minimising untoward effects. Methyldopa also tends to reduce the marked diurnal fluctuations of blood pressure (lowest in the morning and highest in the late afternoon and evening) that often occur with large doses of guanethidine (Leonard et al., 1965).

Dosage: The usual starting dose of guanethidine is 10mg administered once daily; the maintenance dose varies widely among individuals and is generally in the range of 25 to 150mg per day. Because of the cumulative effect of the drug, at least 3 to 5 day intervals should be allowed between changes in dosage. Larger and more frequent increases in dosage are possible in hospitalised patients and Shand has proposed a loading regimen which allows attainment of the maximal pharmacological effect within 4 days (Shand et al., 1975).

Guanethidine should be used with extreme caution in patients with advanced renal insufficiency as gradual accumulation can occur resulting in severe orthostatic hypotension (Gifford, 1973).

Drug Interactions: There are a number of medications which antagonise the effectiveness of guanethidine and related guanidinium compounds (Stone et al., 1964). The tricyclic antidepressants (imipramine, desipramine, nortriptyline, etc), and doxepin at dosages exceeding 200mg daily, competitively block the noradrenaline pump by which guanethidine gains access to the nerve terminal (Mitchell and Oates, 1970; Mitchell et al., 1970; Fann et al., 1971). The administration of these agents therefore results in a gradual rise in blood pressure over several days and this effect persists for about a week after they are withdrawn (Oates et al., 1971). Large doses of guanethidine are required to overcome this antagonism and if the tricyclic agents are suddenly withdrawn without a concomitant decrease in the guanethidine dosage, severe hypotension may result.

Amphetamines also compete for the uptake mechanism (Chang et al., 1965); however, in addition, they also stimulate the release of guanethidine directly from the adrenergic neurone and rapidly reverse the adrenergic blockade (Gulati et al., 1965). Methylphenidate, ephedrine, and to a lesser degree, chlorpromazine also antagonise the antihypertensive effect of guanethidine (Gulati et al., 1965; Gilder et al., 1976), probably by inhibition of the uptake mechanism. Ephedrine is a component of several bronchodilator preparations and 'cold' remedies and is present in sufficient quantities to effectively antagonise the antihypertensive effect of guanethidine (Woosley et al., 1976).

Guanethidine depletes the myocardium of catecholamines and depresses myocardial contractility, and its use in patients with enlarged hearts or a history of congestive heart failure has been questioned (Braunwald et al., 1963). However, the benefit derived from adequate blood pressure control usually more than compensates for the myocardial depressant effect. Great caution should be exercised if guanethidine is used in combination with β-blocking agents as cardiac performance may be seriously impaired (Donald et al., 1965).

Guanethidine is contraindicated in patients with phaeochromocytoma and should not be used in combination with monoamine oxidase (MAO) inhibitors because of the danger of precipitating a hypertensive crisis. Guanethidine therapy is not a contraindication to anaesthesia for elective surgery as long as the anaesthesiologist is aware of denervation hypersensitivity and the importance of maintenance of adequate intravascular volume. The treatment of choice for hypotension as the result of haemorrhage or volume depletion is the Trendelenburg (head-down) position and the infusion of a plasma volume expander such as blood, low molecular weight dextran or isotonic saline. If a pressor agent is required to maintain arterial pressure, indirect acting pressor agents (e.g. ephedrine, metaraminol, etc.) are ineffective because of the depletion of tissue stores of noradrenaline. Direct acting α-agonists such as noradrenaline or phenylephrine are effective in this situation; however, they must be administered cautiously to avoid a hypertensive crisis as a result of the denervation hypersensitivity.

2.2.4 Side Effects

The side effects of guanethidine are usually attributable to excessive sympathetic blockade or unopposed parasympathetic activity. One of the major disadvantages of guanethidine is the orthostatic hypotension it characteristically induces. It occurs most commonly in the morning, when the patient first arises, and improves during the day. Patients must be warned about arising suddenly from the recumbent or seated position. Additional measures such as elastic support stockings and elevating the head of the bed about 15° are also sometimes helpful.

When orthostatic hypotension is a problem, measurement of blood pressure by the patient or a member of his family in the home is indispensable for adequate medical management. Blood pressures should be measured in the supine and standing positions when the patient awakens in the morning and again in the evening. Despite adequate therapy, office pressures are often higher than home pressures. The contrast between postural dizziness and 'resistant hypertension' during office visits, should be carefully evaluated by home recordings before increasing guanethidine therapy.

Exercise hypotension is a relatively common occurrence and can be quite disabling in some patients. It apparently results from a fall in cardiac output due to extensive venous pooling in the lower extremities (Khatri and Cohn, 1970). Elastic support stockings may be of some benefit in this situation.

Diarrhoea resulting from guanethidine therapy is usually most bothersome following meals and in the early morning, when sympathetic activity is normally reduced. It can sometimes be controlled with atropine or related drugs, prescribed according to the patient's pattern of diarrhoea.

Sexual impotence occurs only occasionally with guanethidine; however, male patients frequently notice delayed or retrograde ejaculation (Freis, 1965). Volume expansion, oedema and congestive heart failure can develop in patients with marginal cardiac reserve, although sodium and fluid retention can usually be readily controlled with the appropriate use of diuretic agents.

2.2.5 Bethanidine and Debrisoquine

Bethanidine and debrisoquine are similar to guanethidine in their pharmacological action and appear to be at least as effective, with the same general indications for use. Their antihypertensive effect is of shorter duration than that of guanethidine and both drugs are less likely to cumulate with chronic therapy, thereby enabling dose adjustments to be made more rapidly (see section 2.2.2). Like guanethidine, they may cause orthostatic hypotension, fluid retention and failure of ejaculation, but diarrhoea is not generally a problem with either drug.

Drug interactions with bethanidine and debrisoquine are also similar to those occurring with guanethidine. A so-called monoamine oxidase inhibitor-like 'cheese reaction' has been described with debrisoquine in which a rise in blood pressure occurred in some individuals who consumed cheese during debrisoquine treatment (Amery and Deloof, 1970).

2.3 Rauwolfia Alkaloids

Reserpine, the most widely used derivative of the Rauwolfia alkaloids, is a selective inhibitor of the sympathetic nervous system. Once widely used in the treatment of hypertension, its popularity has waned with the advent of more effective antihypertensive agents with fewer unpleasant side effects.

2.3.1 Mode of Action

Reserpine exerts its sympatholytic effect by depleting the post-ganglionic adrenergic neurones of noradrenaline, and the degree of adrenergic blockade appears to be closely related to the level of noradrenaline depletion (Gaffney et al., 1963). The exact mechanism by which reserpine acts is not completely understood. It is thought, however, that reserpine inhibits the uptake mechanism by which noradrenaline gains entrance into the storage vesicles within the terminal sympathetic nerve endings (Viveros et al., 1969; Haggendal and Dahlstrom, 1972; Shore, 1972; Weiner, 1970), thus exposing it to degradation by cytoplasmic monoamine oxidase (Zarro, 1973; Harrison et al., 1963). Reserpine may also interfere with synthesis of catecholamines by blocking the uptake of dopamine into the storage vesicles where it is enzymatically converted to noradrenaline (Viveros et al., 1969; Rutledge and Weiner, 1967). The noradrenaline pump by which catecholamines gain access to the sympathetic nerve terminal is not inhibited by reserpine (Shore, 1972).

Reserpine rapidly crosses the blood-brain barrier and depletes brain tissue of serotonin and dopamine as well as noradrenaline (Vogt, 1959). This latter action probably accounts for the sedation and depression which is frequently associated with reserpine. However, central sympathetic outflow is not significantly altered by reserpine (Iggo and Vogt, 1960) and the effect on the central nervous system is thought to be less important than its peripheral effect in regard to its antihypertensive potency (Nickerson and Collier, 1975), although this remains controversial.

The reduction in arterial pressure which accompanies the acute administration of reserpine is associated with a reduction in both cardiac output and systemic resistance. With long term therapy, the cardiac output increases to pretreatment levels while the peripheral vascular resistance remains reduced (Sannerstedt and Conway,

1970; Reusch, 1962). Both renal blood flow and glomerular filtration rate are reduced in the early phase of treatment, but both return to pretreatment levels with chronic therapy (Sannerstedt and Conway, 1970; Reusch, 1962; Kisin and Yuzhakov, 1976).

2.3.2 Pharmacokinetics

The Rauwolfia alkaloids are readily absorbed following oral administration (Byck, 1975). Reserpine rapidly disappears from the blood stream and is widely distributed throughout most organ systems including the brain, liver, spleen, kidney and adipose tissue (Carrier, 1972). In the peripheral tissues, reserpine appears to localise within the adrenergic neurones, presumably at the membrane surface of the catecholamine storage vesicles (Shore, 1972).

The metabolic fate of the Rauwolfia compounds has not been completely elucidated; however, it is thought that degradation occurs largely by hydrolysis and demethylation (Domino, 1971). In animal studies, urinary excretion of metabolites occurs within several hours and accounts for about 40% of an orally administered dose, whereas faecal excretion of unchanged reserpine accounts for less than 10% (Aviado, 1972). Whether this is applicable to man remains to be established.

2.3.3 Clinical Use

The usual effective dose ranges from 0.25 to 0.5mg of reserpine per day, although the maintenance dosage should probably not exceed 0.25mg daily in order to minimise side effects (Tarazi and Gifford, 1975; Freis, 1975). A diuretic should be administered concurrently to avoid the possibility of false tolerance (Dustan et al., 1972). Rauwolfia compounds markedly deplete the myocardium of catecholamine stores (Chidsey et al., 1962, 1963) and they have been implicated in aggravating congestive heart failure in certain patients with severely compromised cardiac reserve (Braunwald et al., 1963). However, the benefit derived from reduction of arterial pressure usually more than compensates for any myocardial depressant effect of catecholamine depletion (Tarazi and Gifford, 1975); nevertheless, fluid retention should be prevented with appropriate diuretic therapy.

As with guanethidine and related drugs, Rauwolfia therapy is not a contraindication to anaesthesia for elective surgery (Alper et al., 1963), as long as the anaesthesiologist is forewarned so that blood and fluid replacement will be prompt and adequate in the event of intraoperative hypotension (Tarazi and Gifford, 1975). If a pressor agent is required, direct acting α-adrenoceptor agonists such as noradrenaline or phenylephrine are the drugs of choice (Braunwald et al., 1963), although they must be administered cautiously as denervation hypersensitivity due to catecholamine depletion is to be expected (Tarazi and Gifford, 1975; Fleming and Trendelenburg, 1961).

2.3.4 Side Effects

Excessive sedation, lassitude, depression, bizarre dreams, and nightmares occur frequently and are attributable to the central nervous system effects of Rauwolfia compounds. In one study, depressive reactions occurred in 26 % of the patients treated with reserpine and in 58 % of patients with a previous history of depression (Quetsch et al., 1959). The symptoms of depression often develop insidiously and may be rationalised or go unnoticed. Extrapyramidal symptoms suggestive of a Parkinsonian state occur occasionally. Other side effects encountered include bradycardia, nasal congestion, activation of peptic ulcer and occasionally, diarrhoea and impotence.

Several years ago, reports originating from Britain (Armstrong et al., 1974), Finland (Heinonen et al., 1974) and the Boston Collaborative Drug Surveillance Program in the USA (Jick et al., 1974), suggested an assocation between breast cancer and the use of reserpine-like drugs. Subsequently, additional studies by three independent groups (Mack et al., 1975; Laska et al., 1975; O'Fallon et al., 1975) were unable to demonstrate any relationship between long term treatment with reserpine and an increased incidence of breast cancer. Although some controversy remains, it seems reasonable to conclude that there is at present insufficient evidence to withhold therapy with reserpine because of the purported association with breast malignancy (Editorial, 1975b; Freis, 1975).

2.4 Methyldopa

Since its introduction as an antihypertensive agent over 15 years ago, methyldopa has become one of the most popular sympathetic blocking agents in general use.

2.4.1 Mode of Action

α-Methyldopa was originally conceived as an inhibitor of the enzyme dopa decarboxylase (Sourkes, 1954) and it has been suggested that it produces sympathetic blockade by interfering with the biosynthesis of noradrenaline (Oates et al., 1960). However, subsequent studies have failed to establish a relationship between inhibition of dopa decarboxylase and the reduction of arterial pressure which occurs (Day et al., 1973; Levine and Sjoerdsma, 1964). It has also been proposed that a metabolic product of α-methyldopa, α-methylnoradrenaline, displaces noradrenaline within the post-ganglionic sympathetic nerve endings and acts as a weak or false neurotransmitter substance (Day and Rand, 1964; Cohen, 1966). However, experimental evidence indicates that the antihypertensive effect of methyldopa is not dependent upon blockade of the peripheral sympathetic nervous system (Ayitey-Smith and Varma, 1970; Haefely et al., 1966; Mohammed et al., 1968) and that the vasopressor potency of α-methylnoradrenaline is almost as great as noradrenaline (Altura, 1975; Conradi et al., 1965; Trinker, 1971).

Although the pharmacological mechanism by which methyldopa lowers arterial pressure is not completely understood, there is a growing body of evidence to suggest that the major site of action is within the central nervous system, presumably at the level of the brain stem (Henning, 1969; Van Zwieten, 1976; Henning, 1975; Finch and Haeusler, 1973; Van Zwieten, 1973). Methyldopa readily crosses the blood-brain barrier and is enzymatically converted to α-methylnoradrenaline by dopamine de-carboxylase and β-hydroxydopamine within the adrenergic neurones of the central nervous system (Carlsson and Lindqvist, 1962; Finch and Haeusler, 1973; Conradi et al., 1965). α-Methylnoradrenaline is released with noradrenaline in response to nerve stimulation (Muscholl and Maitre, 1964) and apparently lowers arterial pressure by stimulating central α-adrenoceptors which reduce the sympathetic out-flow from the central nervous system (Heise and Kroneberg, 1972; Baum et al., 1972). Although the mechanism appears complex, current evidence suggests that peripheral adrenergic blockade is probably of secondary importance in regard to the antihypertensive effect of methyldopa (Nickerson and Ruedy, 1975).

The reduction of supine blood pressure with both acute and chronic administra-tion of methyldopa is associated with a fall in systemic vascular resistance and the cardiac output is variably affected but often slightly reduced (Onesti, 1976; Weil et al., 1963; Dollery et al., 1963; Chamberlain and Howard, 1964). In the upright posi-tion, an orthostatic fall in pressure occurs which corresponds to a reduction in cardiac output and little or no change in peripheral resistance (Onesti et al., 1964; Onesti, 1976). Renal blood flow and glomerular filtration rate are maintained (Onesti, 1976; Weil et al., 1963) and myocardial (Cohen et al., 1967) and cerebral blood flow (Meyer et al., 1968) are reported to be increased in many patients.

Like all sympathetic blocking agents (except the β-blockers), methyldopa causes plasma volume expansion and may produce obvious fluid retention and oedema (Weil et al., 1963). Plasma renin activity has been found to be suppressed by some in-vestigators (Mohammed et al., 1969), although this remains somewhat controversial (Lowder and Liddle, 1975).

2.4.2 Pharmacokinetics

Following oral administration of methyldopa 50% or less is absorbed from the gastrointestinal tract, although there is considerable individual variation (range 9 to 75%) [Kwan et al., 1976; Sjoerdsma et al., 1963; Prescott et al., 1966]. Peak plasma levels occur 2 to 6 hours following an oral dose, and methyldopa and its conjugates are rapidly excreted by the kidney (Buhs et al., 1964).

In patients with normal or only mildly impaired renal function, 80 to 90% of the administered dose is eliminated by the kidney within 48 hours, the bulk of it being excreted within 12 hours (Sjoerdsma et al., 1963). In the presence of azotaemia, however, delayed urinary excretion may result in accumulation of methyldopa (Myhre et al., 1972a) and pharmacologically active metabolites such as methyldopa-O-sulphate (Myhre et al., 1972b). Although there is individual variability in absorption, patients who respond appropriately to therapy with methyldopa do not differ significantly in regard to gastrointestinal absorption from those who do not (Au et al., 1972; Prescott et al., 1966).

2.4.3 Clinical Use

Methyldopa is a sympatholytic agent of moderate potency. Following oral or intravenous administration, it has a delayed onset of action (2 to 3 hours) and its maximum antihypertensive effect occurs 5 to 10 hours following administration. The usual starting dose is 250mg 2 or 3 times daily and this may be increased to 2g or more per day. Little additional therapeutic benefit is derived from doses above this level. Methyldopa should be used in combination with an appropriate diuretic agent to prevent the development of false tolerance due to plasma volume expansion (Dustan et al., 1972). The combination of a diuretic and methyldopa is often effective in controlling mild to moderate hypertension which has not responded optimally to diuretics alone.

Methyldopa and its metabolites interfere with the fluorescent technique for determining catecholamines and may cause false elevations of plasma and urinary catecholamines which could be misconstrued as evidence of phaeochromocytoma.

2.4.4 Side Effects

Among the most commonly encountered side effects are somnolence, dry mouth, nasal congestion, orthostatic hypotension and impotence. Approximately 20 % of patients receiving methyldopa develop a positive direct Coombs' test, yet haemolytic anaemia is rare (Carstairs et al., 1966; Worlledge et al., 1966). In the absence of anaemia, the positive direct Coombs' test is not a contraindication to continuation of therapy; however, the haematocrit should be checked periodically (Surveyor et al., 1968). Drug fever (Glontz and Saslaw, 1968) and drug induced hepatitis (Elkington et al., 1969; Miller and Reid, 1976) have been observed in a few patients receiving methyldopa.

A reversible form of dementia has been reported to occur when haloperidol was used in combination with methyldopa (Thornton, 1976). A hypertensive crisis has been attributed to the intravenous administration of propranolol in one patient receiving methyldopa (Nies and Shand, 1973).

Although clinical data are sparse (White, 1965), pharmacological data from animal studies suggest that the tricyclic antidepressants may interfere with the antihypertensive effect of methyldopa (Kale and Satoskar, 1970; Van Zwieten, 1977). However, this interaction has been questioned (Briant et al., 1973) and requires further evaluation.

2.5 Clonidine

2.5.1 Mode of Action

Clonidine is a centrally acting sympatholytic agent with antihypertensive potency comparable to that of methyldopa (Putzeys and Hoobler, 1972). Pharmacologically, clonidine is an α-adrenoceptor agonist and lowers blood pressure by stimulation of post-synaptic α-adrenoceptors in the vasomotor centres of the medulla
(Haeusler, 1975; Kobinger, 1976). This results in inhibition of sympathetic outflow
from the central nervous system and enhanced vagal stimulation, which presumably
results from facilitation of the pressure sensitive baroreceptor reflex by the action of
clonidine (Kobinger, 1975, 1976).

The haemodynamic changes which occur with clonidine consist of a fall in arterial pressure which is associated with a decrease in heart rate and cardiac output
with little or no change in systemic resistance (Onesti et al., 1969, 1971). Because it
does not interfere with the baroreceptor reflex, clonidine does not usually produce a
marked orthostatic change in pressure and exercise hypotension is uncommon (Lund-
Johansen, 1976). The renal blood flow and glomerular filtration rate are maintained
as there is a reduction in renal vascular resistance (Onesti et al., 1969). Clonidine sup-
presses renin secretion, possibly by a centrally mediated decrease in renal sympathetic
neural tone (Reid et al., 1975).

2.5.2 Pharmacokinetics

Clonidine is well absorbed from the gastrointestinal tract and 65 to 90% is excreted in the urine within 72 hours following oral administration (Conolly, 1975;
Rehbinder and Deckers, 1969). Peak plasma levels appear within 2 to 4 hours and
clonidine disappears from the plasma with a half-life of 12 hours in patients with normal renal function (Dollery et al., 1975). The plasma levels of clonidine have been
found to correlate well with the pharmacological effects including the lowering of
recumbent blood pressure, sedation and decrease in salivary flow (Dollery et al.,
1975). In patients with diminished renal function, the pharmacokinetics of clonidine
remain to be clarified.

2.5.3 Clinical Use

Intravenous administration of clonidine is immediately associated with a transient increase in blood pressure of several minutes duration, followed by a gradual
reduction of pressure which lasts for several hours. This transient pressor response is
apparently due to direct stimulation of peripheral α-adrenoceptors by clonidine and
can be prevented by pretreatment with the α-adrenoceptor antagonist, phenoxybenzamine (Bock et al., 1973).

Following oral administration, the maximal antihypertensive effect occurs after
2 to 4 hours and persists for 6 to 10 hours (Onesti et al., 1969). The usual starting
dose is 0.1 mg twice daily and this may be gradually increased to as much as 0.6 mg 3

or 4 times daily. Clonidine produces sodium and water retention with expansion of the plasma and extracellular fluid volume, which counteracts its antihypertensive effect. It should, therefore, be combined with an oral diuretic agent; it is best used for the management of mild to moderate hypertension which has not responded adequately to treatment with a diuretic alone.

2.5.4 Side Effects

The adverse effects associated with clonidine therapy include drowsiness (which may be severe in some patients), dryness of the mouth, constipation, and fluid retention. Symptomatic orthostatic hypotension is rarely encountered (Pettinger, 1975).

The sudden cessation of therapy with clonidine can result in a withdrawal syndrome with 'rebound hypertension' and symptoms of restlessness, agitation, nausea, sweating and insomnia. Presumably, this is mediated by hyperactivity of the sympathetic nervous system with excessive catecholamine release (Hansson et al., 1973) and can be reversed by reinstituting therapy with clonidine and then withdrawing it gradually (Pettinger, 1975). In the event of a crisis, the blood pressure can be reduced by the administration of an α-adrenoceptor blocking agent such as phentolamine and, if necessary, tachycardia can be controlled by the careful addition of a β-adrenoreceptor blocking agent such as propranolol (Kosman, 1975; Goldberg et al., 1976; Harris, 1976). The frequency of the clonidine withdrawal reactions has probably been over-rated; however, loss of blood pressure control following cessation of clonidine seems to be unusually rapid. The intensity of the rebound phenomenon has been chiefly correlated with the dose of clonidine used (Goldberg et al., 1976) and seems less dramatic with short term therapy (Hanson et al., 1973). Patients receiving clonidine should be instructed about the hazard of abruptly discontinuing treatment.

β-Blockade has been reported to exaggerate the 'rebound hypertension' that sometimes accompanies the sudden withdrawal of clonidine (Bailey and Neale, 1976). The tricyclic antidepressants may antagonise the antihypertensive effect of clonidine in some patients (Briant et al., 1973; Van Zwieten, 1975).

2.6 Prazosin

2.6.1 Mode of Action

Prazosin is a relatively new peripheral vasodilator antihypertensive agent. Pharmacologically, it is a quinazoline derivative and an inhibitor of the enzyme phosphodiesterase which hydrolyses cyclic-AMP and cyclic-GMP (Hess, 1974). Its mechanism of action is not yet fully understood. It was originally thought to have a direct relaxant effect on arteriolar smooth muscle, presumably by increasing intracellular cyclic-AMP (Hess, 1974), but it has now been shown to have α-adrenoceptor blocking properties (Graham et al., 1977). Experimental evidence suggests that its mode of action probably resides in selective interference with post-synaptic α-adrenoceptors

(Wood et al., 1975; Bolli et al., 1975). Unlike conventional α-adrenoceptor blocking drugs, it has little or no affinity for pre-synaptic α-receptors (Cambridge et al.,
1977).

The antihypertensive action of prazosin is usually not associated with a reflex increase in heart rate or cardiac output and it does not stimulate renin secretion (Hayes
et al., 1976; Graham et al., 1976; Koshy et al., 1977). Its pharmacological effect occurs at the level of the resistance vessels as well as the venous capacitance vessels
(Awan et al., 1977). Following acute and chronic administration, prazosin lowers arterial pressure by decreasing peripheral vascular resistance and cardiac output is
usually unchanged or slightly increased (Lund-Johansen, 1975). Because of the relaxant effect on venous capacitance vessels, prazosin may cause a reduction in venous
return to the heart. Therefore, prazosin may reduce cardiac preload and afterload and
has been reported to improve left ventricular performance in patients with refractory
heart failure, even when hypertension is minimal or absent (Miller et al., 1977; Awan
et al., 1978). Renal blood flow and glomerular filtration rate are maintained with
prazosin (Koshy et al., 1977). Fluid retention may occur in some patients and reduce
its antihypertensive potency (Koshy et al., 1977).

2.6.2 Pharmacokinetics

The pharmacokinetics of prazosin are not well understood. It appears to be well
absorbed from the gastrointestinal tract (Brogden et al., 1977) and peak plasma concentrations occur within 2 to 3 hours (Wood et al., 1976); however, its therapeutic
action does not appear to be closely related with plasma levels (Collins and Pek,
1975).

Following absorption in animals, prazosin is rapidly distributed throughout
most tissues, and it appears to have a predilection for blood vessels (Hess, 1974).
Animal studies have shown that prazosin is extensively metabolised by the liver and
is predominantly excreted via the biliary tract (Wood et al., 1976). Higher and more
prolonged serum levels of the drug have been reported in patients with renal insufficiency (Brogden et al., 1977).

2.6.3 Clinical Use

Prazosin is an antihypertensive agent of modest potency comparable with that of
methyldopa (Venables and Duff, 1974), clonidine and reserpine. Following oral administration, the maximum antihypertensive effect occurs within 4 to 5 hours and its
therapeutic action persists for about 10 hours (Collins and Pek, 1975). The usual
starting dosage of 0.5mg tablets twice daily or 1mg capsules 2 or 3 times daily[1] can
be increased by increments at weekly intervals as necessary to a maximum of 10mg 2

---

1 The initial dosage with the capsules (available in the USA) is higher as lower peak plasma levels
are said to be attained with this dose form than with the tablets (available in other countries).

or 3 times daily. When it is used by itself, approximately 80% of patients with mild to moderate hypertension will have a significant fall in pressure, although a delayed onset of maximum effect (2 to 14 weeks) has been observed (Bolzano, 1974).

Prazosin should be used in combination with a diuretic as the therapeutic action is enhanced (Lund-Johansen, 1975) and plasma volume expansion, which may occur in some patients, is effectively controlled (Koshy et al., 1977). Because of its α-adrenoceptor blocking properties, it could be used as an alternative to one of the sympathetic inhibiting agents in step 2 of table IV (see section 5). It has also been used successfully in combination with sympathetic inhibiting drugs and may be used as an alternative to hydrallazine in step 3 of table IV. Prazosin is also effective in the management of patients with renal insufficiency and is often effective in relatively low doses (Bolzano, 1974; Curtis and Bateman, 1975).

Orthostatic hypotension not uncommonly occurs at the onset of treatment but this usually disappears with continued therapy (Bolzano, 1974). Reports of syncopal episodes occurring within 30 to 90 minutes following the initial dose of prazosin have led to the introduction of the term 'first-dose effect'. These episodes have been attributed to the development of marked orthostatic hypotension and have been estimated to occur in at least 1% of patients (Editorial, 1975a). Present evidence suggests that the 'first-dose effect' may be more severe in patients who are receiving β-adrenoceptor blocking drugs or who may be relatively depleted of sodium as a result of previous diuretic therapy. However, its occurrence can be largely avoided by beginning treatment with a low dose (0.5mg tablets twice daily or 1mg capsules 2 or 3 times daily) and giving the first dose at bedtime (Brogden et al., 1977; Turner et al., 1977). Patients who experience orthostatic symptoms with prazosin may tolerate reinstitution of therapy at a lower dose without difficulty if the dose is reduced to 0.5mg once or twice daily (Turner et al., 1975). Whether such symptoms differ significantly from those seen with other neuroplegic agents or warrant a special term is indeed questionable.

2.6.4 Side Effects

Prazosin is generally well tolerated and is associated with a relatively low incidence of untoward reactions. Headache, palpitation, drowsiness, dizziness, and orthostatic hypotension are the most common adverse effects. Sexual disturbances which are relatively common with many other antihypertensive agents are rare with prazosin.

2.7 β-Adrenoceptor Blocking Agents (β-Blockers)

Since 1964, when Prichard described the reduction of arterial pressure with pronethalol, β-adrenoceptor blocking agents have become increasingly popular as antihypertensive agents. Propranolol was the first β-blocking agent to come into general

Table III. Pharmacological properties of β-adrenoceptor blocking drugs (after Waal-Manning, 1976)

Drug	β-Blockade potency ratio (propranolol = 1)	Cardio-selectivity	Partial agonist activity	Membrane stabilising activity
Acebutolol	0.3	+	+	+
Alprenolol	0.3	0	+ +	+
Atenolol	1	+	0	0
Metoprolol	1	+	0	±
Oxprenolol	0.5–1	0	+ +	+
Pindolol (prindolol)	6	0	+ + +	+
Practolol	0.3	+	+ +	0
Propranolol	1	0	0	+ +
Sotalol	0.3	0	0	0
Timolol	6	0	±	0
Isomer: d-propanolol	0.1	0	0	+ +

use and its success prompted the development and introduction of a number of similar agents such as practolol, alprenolol, oxprenolol, timolol, acebutolol and others. Because of their effectiveness and relative freedom from irritating side effects, these agents have gained wide acceptance as first-line drugs in the treatment of hypertension.

The currently available β-blocking agents and their pharmacological properties are listed in table III. These drugs act by competitively inhibiting the effects of catecholamines at β-adrenoceptor sites, and their pharmacological potencies are determined by their relative abilities to inhibit isoprenaline-induced tachycardia. The various agents are often classified according to their organ sensitivities. Acebutolol[2], atenolol, metoprolol and practolol are often referred to as 'cardioselective agents' as they are 50 to 100 times more potent in inhibiting cardiac β-adrenoceptors (β_1-receptors) than the receptors of the peripheral vasculature and bronchial smooth muscle (β_2-receptors) [Waal-Manning, 1976]. The other agents are relatively 'non-selective' in regard to their activities against β_1 and β_2-adrenoceptors. However, the

2 The cardioselectivity of acebutolol has been disputed by some authorities (Dollery, 1973; Shanks, personal communications). However, acebutolol has recently been shown to exhibit significant cardioselectivity in man, although it is less cardioselective than practolol (Wollam et al., 1978).

separation is obviously not absolute, as inhibition of vascular or bronchial receptors occurs when the concentrations of the so-called 'cardioselective agents' is high enough. For example, low serum concentrations of practolol (0.9µg/ml) produced 40% blockade of heart rate response to exercise but did not alter forearm vasodilatation in response to isoprenaline. In contrast, high serum concentrations of practolol (5.9µg/ml) were associated with equal blockade of both cardiac and vascular responses (Lertora et al., 1975).

Several of the β-blocking agents exhibit a small but measurable agonist response when exposed to β-adrenoceptors in the absence of a primary β-agonist such as isoprenaline or adrenaline. This partial agonistic property has been termed 'intrinsic sympathomimetic activity' and is characteristic of acebutolol, alprenolol, oxprenolol, pindolol and practolol. The other β-blocking agents, propranolol, sotalol, timolol, atenolol, and metoprolol have no measurable agonist effect (Imhof, 1975). Current evidence suggests, however, that relative differences in potency, 'cardioselectivity', intrinsic sympathomimetic activity and membrane stabilising properties are probably of little significance in determining the antihypertensive effectiveness of the various β-blocking drugs (Hansson and Werko, 1977; Niarchos and Tarazi, 1976; Nies and Shand, 1975). In spite of known differences in pharmacological activity, most of the drugs seem to induce similar antihypertensive responses if administered in appropriate doses. Moreover, patients who fail to respond to one β-blocking agent generally fail to respond to the others (Waal-Manning, 1976; Morgan et al., 1974; Doyle, 1974).

2.7.1 Mode of Action

Early studies of the blood pressure lowering effect of propranolol demonstrated a chronic reduction in cardiac output with essentially no change in the total peripheral resistance. This led to the initial suggestion that the antihypertensive effect of propranolol was primarily related to the reduction in cardiac output (Lydtin et al., 1972). It was therefore speculated that β-blockade might be most effective in those hypertensive patients with an increased cardiac output. However, recent studies have revealed a more complex mechanism in regard to the blood pressure lowering effect of β-blocking agents, and haemodynamic parameters have been found to be of little value in predicting the response to β-blockade (Tarazi and Dustan, 1972; Tarazi et al., 1976).

A striking contrast exists between the immediate and long term haemodynamic effects of β-adrenoceptor blockade with propranolol (Niarchos and Tarazi, 1976). Whereas the cardiac output is depressed to the same extent by acute intravenous or chronic oral administration of propranolol, arterial pressure is reduced only with long term treatment (Tarazi, 1973b; Frohlich et al., 1968). The antihypertensive action of propranolol is therefore apparently related to the adaptability of peripheral resistance to long term reductions in flow. With the chronic oral administration of propranolol, as with other β-blocking drugs, the arterial pressure response correlates best with changes in peripheral resistance and not at all with variations in cardiac output or heart rate (Nies and Shand, 1975).

The importance of total peripheral resistance in determining the blood pressure response to β-blockade is underscored by the observations that some β-blockers may reduce blood pressure without reducing cardiac output (Niarchos and Tarazi, 1976; Franciosa and Freis, 1975; Franciosa et al., 1973). This concept also explains the failure of propranolol to control transient pressor responses associated with painful· stimuli or with mental or emotional stress. The increase in heart rate and cardiac output normally responsible for these blood pressure elevations has been shown to be effectively blocked by propranolol; however, the rise in arterial pressure still occurs in response to stressful stimuli as the result of an increase in total peripheral resistance. Administration of propranolol merely alters the haemodynamic mechanism responsible for the rise in pressure from an increase in cardiac output to a rise in peripheral resistance (Tarazi and Dustan, 1972; Tarazi et al., 1976).

In regard to the antihypertensive mechanisms of the other β-blocking agents, an extensive literature has developed describing their various haemodynamic features. As a general rule, however, the reduction in cardiac output is usually less pronounced than with propranolol and readjustments in peripheral resistance generally occur more rapidly (Niarchos and Tarazi, 1976). Our own experience has been mainly with practolol. Although the long term clinical use of practolol has recently been discontinued because of serious ocular, cutaneous and peritoneal complications, the earlier haemodynamic experience with this agent has been useful in furthering our understanding of the antihypertensive effect of β-adrenoceptor blockade. The immediate effects of practolol on heart rate, cardiac output and peripheral vascular resistance were similar to those of propranolol, but the long term haemodynamic effect was substantially different in that cardiac output was often increased rather than lowered by oral practolol and peripheral resistance was reduced below pretreatment levels (Niarchos and Tarazi, 1976).

Sannerstedt (1975) has reviewed the haemodynamic effect of several β-blocking agents. He concluded that the haemodynamic pattern was consistently characterised by an initial reduction of heart rate and cardiac output which is accompanied by an elevation of total peripheral resistance that may gradually decrease with chronic administration. As stressed by many authors, the extent of these effects is not uniform but may vary according to the presence or absence of cardioselectivity and intrinsic sympathomimetic activity, as well as to differences in pre-blockade haemodynamic patterns and differences in duration of therapy.

Some observers have suggested that the blood pressure response to propranolol is closely correlated with both the pretreatment level of plasma renin activity and the magnitude of renin suppression produced (Buhler et al., 1972). These results seemed to suggest that hypertensive patients with hyperreninaemia have good responses to treatment with propranolol and that patients with suppressed renin levels respond poorly. Although it is well established that renin secretion by the kidneys is at least partially mediated by adrenergic receptors, and that renin release can be inhibited in certain circumstances by propranolol, there is a growing body of evidence to suggest a dissociation between the reduction in plasma renin activity and the lowering of arterial pressure. A number of studies have failed to demonstrate a significant correlation between the fall in blood pressure and the reduction in plasma renin activity (Bravo et al., 1974, 1975a,b; Anavekar et al., 1975; Woods et al., 1976; Mookerjee et al., 1977); moreover, relatively low doses of propranolol are required to suppress plasma renin activity, whereas substantially larger doses are required to lower blood pressure (Michelakis and McAllister, 1972). There are also major differences among the various β-blocking agents in regard to suppression of renin release. For example, pindolol, when given acutely, causes considerable reduction in blood pressure with little or no obvious effect on the level of plasma renin activity (Morgan et al., 1975). The evidence therefore suggests that there is probably no significant relationship between the suppression of renin release and the antihypertensive effect of the β-blocking agents (Bravo et al., 1975b; Michelakis and McAllister, 1972).

It has also been suggested that β-blocking agents may lower blood pressure via a central nervous mechanism, possibly similar to that of clonidine and methyldopa. This suggestion is supported by the observation that the injection of propranolol directly into the cerebral ventricles of experimental animals rapidly produces hypotension (Lewis, 1975). Moreover, highly lipid soluble drugs such as propranolol equilibrate rapidly between CNS and plasma, and high concentrations of propranolol have been found within the brain tissue of patients receiving the drug who have come to autopsy (Waal-Manning, 1976; Myers et al., 1975). The clinical observation that many of the β-blockers produce side effects such as sedation, vivid dreams, hallucinations and occasional depression, further strengthens the hypothesis that these agents have definite sites of action within the CNS (Waal, 1967; Simpson, 1974). This concept is far from proven, however, because other β-blockers such as practolol enter the brain poorly, yet have been shown to lower blood pressure.

2.7.2 Pharmacokinetics

All the β-blocking agents with the possible exception of atenolol, are well absorbed from the alimentary tract following oral administration (Johnsson and Regardh, 1976; Shand, 1974). Peak blood levels generally occur within 1 to 3 hours; however, for most β-blockers there is a lag time between maximum blood levels, and maximum antihypertensive effect. This is probably a reflection of the time required to reach tissue receptors and may in part explain why there have been conflicting reports on the correlation between plasma levels and the antihypertensive effect (Johnsson and Regardh, 1976; Waal-Manning, 1976). Although most β-blockers have a relatively short plasma half-life, the duration of the antihypertensive effect is relatively long lasting and persists up to 24 hours or longer for some agents (Carruthers et al., 1973). A correlation between the plasma level and therapeutic effect has been demonstrated for alprenolol (Collste et al., 1976), propranolol (Cleaveland and

Shand, 1971), sotalol (Sundquist et al., 1974) and pindolol (Anavekar et al., 1975; Waal-Manning, 1976), but studies thus far have failed to demonstrate a significant correlation for metoprolol (Bengtsson et al., 1974), oxprenolol (Brunner et al., 1975), and practolol (Sundquist et al., 1974). The difference in the time-course between the antihypertensive effect and the plasma level means that for most β-blockers a twice daily (or in some cases once daily) dosage regimen can be used.

With most β-blockers there seems to be a ceiling dose above which increasing the dose does not lead to a greater antihypertensive response (Waal-Manning, 1976). An exception to this is propranolol for example for which doses as high as 4g per day have been employed in some patients. This is due to the fact that propranolol is subject to considerable first-pass hepatic metabolism, and because of the very great variation in the extent of this phenomenon between individuals, very high doses may be needed in some cases to obtain a response. However, taking them as a group, it remains controversial whether such large doses of propranolol lead to better overall control of blood pressure in hypertensive patients (Lydtin et al., 1972).

In regard to metabolism and excretion of the various β-blocking agents, propranolol and alprenolol are eliminated almost entirely by hepatic degradation, whereas practolol and sotalol are eliminated largely by renal mechanisms (Johnsson and Regardh, 1976; Shand, 1974). Metoprolol is mainly excreted by the kidneys following biotransformation, while pindolol, acebutolol, atenolol and timolol are eliminated to a variable extent by both routes (Johnsson and Regardh, 1976; Waal-Manning, 1976). The plasma half-lives of drug such as practolol and sotalol which are eliminated mainly by renal mechanisms are markedly prolonged in the presence of renal failure. Similarly, the plasma half-lives of those drugs whose primary mode of elimination is by hepatic degradation are prolonged in the presence of liver disease, and also in uraemia, which has been shown to decrease first-pass hepatic metabolism of propranolol and probably also alprenolol (Johnsson and Regardh, 1976; Waal-Manning, 1976a). One should be aware of the possible accumulation of active metabolites of propranolol and alprenolol in patients with severe chronic renal insufficiency not undergoing regular dialysis (Waal-Manning, 1976; Bianchett et al., 1976) and of the decreased first-pass metabolism of oral labetalol (increased bioavailability) in chronic liver disease (Homeida et al., 1978).

2.7.3 Clinical Use

β-Adrenoceptor blocking agents are increasing in popularity as antihypertensive agents, not only because of their effectiveness in lowering blood pressure, but also because they are exceptionally well tolerated by most patients. They rarely cause orthostatic hypotension and are usually not associated with disturbances in sexual potency (Zacharias et al., 1972; Simpson, 1974). Only infrequently are they associated with sedation or depression such as often occurs with reserpine, methyldopa or clonidine. In several studies conducted on large groups of patients in which β-blockers were employed in combination with other drugs and their contraindications carefully respected, approximately 85 % of patients treated reported no noticeable side effects (Hansson and Werko, 1977; Zacharias et al., 1972). In the vast majority of studies performed thus far, the development of side effects necessitating discontinuation of treatment has been a relatively uncommon occurrence.

When used by themselves, β-blocking agents produce a significant reduction in arterial pressure in only about 30 % of the patients, and the fall in pressure generally occurs gradually over a period of several weeks (Morgan et al., 1974; Tarazi and Dustan, 1972). However, when employed in combined regimens with other antihypertensive agents, especially with diuretics and vasodilators, an additive antihypertensive effect is generally obtained, and a satisfactory reduction in blood pressure can usually be achieved in 80 % or more of patients (Zacharias et al., 1972). β-Blocking agents have been used to prevent the reflex tachycardia of hydrallazine (Sannerstedt et al., 1971; Sannerstedt et al., 1972) and they are superior to reserpine, methyldopa or guanethidine in this role. Conversely, hydrallazine and other vasodilators such as prazosin prevent the initial rise in peripheral resistance induced by the β-blocking agents, and the combination of a β-blocking agent and a vasodilator, usually with a diuretic, has been effective in managing moderate and severe hypertension (Zacest et al., 1972; Goble, 1975; Marshall et al., 1977).

The evidence indicates that the various β-blocking agents have similar antihypertensive activity when administered in appropriate dosages to allow for differences in their pharmacological potencies. Patients responding to one β-blocking drug generally respond in similar fashion to other agents and conversely, patients who fail to respond to one β-blocking agent, generally fail to respond to others (Morgan et al., 1974). The β-adrenoceptor blocking agents can be especially useful in the following circumstances:

1) *Patients with coexisting angina pectoris.* In this setting the β-blocking drugs are ideal agents because of their known effectiveness in treating angina pectoris. However, they should not be discontinued abruptly in patients with known coronary disease since exacerbations of myocardial ischaemia have been reported under these circumstances.

2) *Patients with certain cardiac arrhythmias.* β-Blocking agents are often effective in treating both supraventricular and ventricular arrhythmias in the absence of cardiac conduction disturbances.

3) *Patients on tricyclic antidepressants and antipsychotic agents.* Whereas the antihypertensive effect of guanethidine is antagonised by phenothiazines and tricyclic antidepressants (nortriptyline, desipramine, protriptyline, etc.), no such effect is noted with the β-blocking agents. However, caution is advised in their use in mentally disturbed patients as depression and even suicide have been described in association with propranolol (Simpson, 1974).

4) *Patients in whom postural hypotension may be dangerous.* As discussed previously, the β-blockers do not cause postural hypotension.

5) *Patients with hyperkinetic essential hypertension.* Hypertensives with a hyperkinetic circulatory state have an increased cardiac output and often suffer from disturbing palpitations and tachycardia. It has been shown that propranolol is often useful in ameliorating the cardiac symptoms in such cases; however, it does not necessarily control the hypertension.

2.7.4 Side Effects

There are a number of potentially serious side effects which are occasionally associated with β-adrenoceptor blocking agents. Patients with a history of bronchial asthma or obstructive airway disease should probably not receive β-blockers because of the possibility of aggravating bronchospasm. Presumably, the 'cardioselective' agents (because of their lesser affinity for the β_2 receptors) and the agents with 'intrinsic sympathomimetic activity' (because of their partial agonistic effect) should have less tendency to produce bronchospasm. However, these considerations are probably more theoretical than practical. Although some high risk patients receiving bronchodilator therapy may do well with cautious use of the so-called 'cardioselective drugs', these agents do have the potential for precipitating bronchospasm, especially at higher dosages, and should be avoided if at all possible (Beumer, 1974).

In general, β-blocking agents should not be administered to patients with bradycardia or those with atrioventricular conduction disturbances. The aggravation or precipitation of congestive heart failure in patients with serious cardiac disease occurs occasionally, but appears to be a relatively infrequent complication. β-Blockade can mask the warning symptoms of hypoglycaemia and can inhibit the release of glycogen, thus prolonging the duration of hypoglycaemia. For these reasons, β-blockers should be given cautiously, if at all, to insulin-dependent brittle diabetics. Central nervous system side effects including hallucinations, bizarre dreams, nightmares, insomnia and depression seem to be especially common with several of the β-blocking agents including propranolol and pindolol (Waal-Manning, 1976a).

A serious immunological disturbance, the so-called 'oculomucocutaneous syndrome' has been associated with the administration of practolol and has led to curtailment of its use. The syndrome affects the eyes, skin, mucous and serous membranes and is sometimes associated with a positive antinuclear factor (Editorial, 1975c; Waal-Manning, 1976a). The syndrome is usually reversible upon withdrawal of practolol, although polyserositis and fibrosing peritonitis may continue to progress despite its discontinuation.

Aggravation of arterial insufficiency has been observed in patients with peripheral arterial occlusive disease (Frohlich et al., 1969), and worsening of renal insufficiency has been reported in a few patients (Swainson and Winney, 1976; Warren et al., 1974; Thompson and Joekes, 1974; Ibsen and Sederberg-Olsen, 1973; Warren, 1976). There is a growing body of evidence to suggest that certain β-blocking agents, such as propranolol, may aggravate glucose intolerance in some patients (Waal-Manning, 1976b), and precipitation of hyperosmolar coma has been reported rarely (Podolsky and Pattavina, 1973). Although the exact mechanism has not been elucidated, there is some evidence to suggest that suppression of insulin release may play a role (Cerasi et al., 1972; Myers and Hope-Gill, 1977; Blum et al., 1975). However, this remains to be clarified. A paradoxical hypertensive crisis has been observed on one occasion when propranolol was administered intravenously to a patient receiving therapy with methyldopa (Nies and Shand, 1973). This unusual occurrence was presumably due to enhanced α-agonistic activity of the metabolite of methyldopa, α-methylnoradrenaline, in the presence of β-adrenoceptor blockade (Nies and Shand, 1973).

A paradoxical rise in blood pressure has also been reported in patients receiving high doses of pindolol; Waal-Manning and Simpson (1975) have described 9 patients in whom blood pressure fell when the dose of pindolol was reduced from a mean of 48mg daily to 19mg daily.

2.8 Labetalol

This recently introduced drug has both α- and β-adrenoceptor blocking properties. The α-blocking effect is relatively less than that of the β-blocking effect, the ratio of the two effects (α:β) after oral administration being approximately 1 : 3. Like propranolol, labetalol is 'non-selective' with respect to β-adrenoceptors and lacks 'intrinsic sympathomimetic activity' (Richards, 1976). However, unlike propranolol and the β-blocking drugs generally, acute administration of labetalol reduces blood pressure and peripheral vascular resistance with no consistent effect on cardiac output (Koch, 1972; Prichard et al., 1975). During long term oral administration, heart rate is consistently reduced but cardiac output is only reduced during exercise (Edwards and Raftery, 1976).

Therapeutic trials have shown labetalol to be effective in lowering blood pressure in hypertension of all grades of severity (Kane et al., 1976; Prichard and Boakes, 1976; Bolli et al., 1976). In mild to moderate hypertension, the drug is generally effective at doses of 300 to 800mg daily, but much higher doses (1.2 to 4g or more daily) are necessary in severe and resistant cases. Labetalol has also been used intravenously for rapid reduction of severely elevated blood pressure, including cases of phaeochromocytoma and clonidine withdrawal hypertension (Rosei et al., 1976; Rønne-Rasmussen et al., 1976). Results with intravenous labetalol have been less satisfactory in severely hypertensive patients receiving concomitant therapy with combinations of various other antihypertensive drugs such as β-adrenoceptor blockers, clonidine, α-methyldopa and bethanidine or debrisoquine (Anderson and Gabriel, 1978; MacCarthy et al., 1978). The most significant side effect of labetalol is posture-related dizziness, which in some instances has been associated with postural hypotension. This effect tends to occur more frequently with higher dosages (above 800mg daily) and early in the course of treatment (Kane et al., 1976; Dargie et al., 1976).

The place of this agent in the treatment of hypertension has still to be adequately defined. Since it has α-blocking properties in addition to a β-blocking effect, labetalol theoretically offers some advantages over conventional β-blockers but any real advantage, particularly in mild or moderate hypertension, has yet to be conclusively demonstrated. It may prove most useful in patients who are not responding adequately to a combined β-blocker/diuretic regimen.

2.9 MAO Inhibitors

Because of their potentially dangerous side effects, the monoamine oxidase inhibitors are seldom used nowadays with the advent of newer sympatholytic agents with fewer side effects. Pargyline is the only commercially available MAO inhibitor for the treatment of hypertension. It is a potent antihypertensive agent which, like guanethidine, selectively blocks sympathetic transmission by preventing the release of noradrenaline at the neuroeffector junction (Puig et al., 1972). Although the exact relationship of MAO inhibition to its antihypertensive action is unclear, it is hypothesised that there is an accumulation of dopamine and octopamine, which may function as false neurotransmitters (Kopin et al., 1965) or interfere with the biosynthesis of noradrenaline (Nickerson and Ruedy, 1975).

Like other MAO inhibitors, pargyline causes an accumulation of noradrenaline within the sympathetic nerve terminal as degradation by monoamine oxidase is markedly reduced. Such an accumulation may cause a potentially fatal drug interaction with agents such as tyramine, ephedrine or amphetamines. These agents cause the release of noradrenaline stores producing a severe hypertensive crisis which must be treated promptly with intravenous phentolamine to prevent a catastrophe. Certain foods (pickled herring, aged cheeses, chicken livers) and beverages (Chianti wine, some naturally fermented beers) contain enough tyramine to trigger this reaction. For this reason the use of pargyline is potentially dangerous and should be discouraged.

3. Direct-acting Vasodilators

3.1 Hydrallazine

3.1.1 Mode of Action
Hydrallazine is a peripheral vasodilator of moderate antihypertensive potency. It exerts its antihypertensive action by producing vasodilatation of the precapillary resistance vessels by direct relaxation of the arteriolar smooth muscle (Stunkard et al., 1954). Hydrallazine has little or no effect on postcapillary venous capacitance vessels (Ablad and Johnsson, 1963).

The cellular mechanism by which hydrallazine acts is not well understood. However, it may be related to the ability of hydrallazine to chelate trace metals which may be required for smooth muscle contraction (Moyer and Brest, 1961; Perry, 1953). The peripheral vasodilatation which occurs with hydrallazine is widespread but not uniform, as vascular resistance is reduced to a greater extent in the splanchnic and renal circulation than in skin and skeletal muscle (Freis et al., 1953). Hydrallazine exerts no appreciable effect on non-vascular smooth muscle and has no direct effect on the myocardium (Koch-Weser, 1974).

The decrease in arterial pressure which accompanies the administration of hydrallazine is associated with a reduction of peripheral resistance and a reflex increase in heart rate, stroke volume, and cardiac output (Rowe et al., 1955). This hydrallazine-induced hyperkinetic circulatory state is due to activation of the baroreceptor reflex by the lowering of blood pressure, resulting in increased adrenergic stimulation to the heart (Chidsey and Gottlieb, 1974). The increase in cardiac output reduces the antihypertensive effect of hydrallazine and is responsible for many of its side effects.

With acute administration, renal blood flow is increased (Judson et al., 1956; Wilkinson et al., 1952). However, it returns to pretreatment levels with chronic administration (Vanderkolk et al., 1954). The glomerular filtration rate is not significantly altered and for this reason, hydrallazine may have no particular advantage in the management of patients with diminished renal function (Moyer and Brest, 1961). Hydrallazine causes sodium and fluid retention with expansion of the plasma and extracellular fluid volumes, and this counteracts its antihypertensive effect (Finnerty, 1971). Peripheral renin activity is increased with hydrallazine therapy, possibly as a result of increased sympathetic discharge (Ueda et al., 1970). The combination of high cardiac output, elevated renin and hypervolaemia may limit or thwart the antihypertensive effectiveness of hydrallazine and this explains the therapeutic efficacy of its combination with diuretics and β-blocking agents.

3.1.2 Pharmacokinetics

Following oral administration, hydrallazine is rapidly and almost completely absorbed (65 to 90 %) and less than 10 % of an oral dose is excreted in the faeces (Lesser et al., 1973, 1974). Peak plasma concentrations occur within one hour (Talseth, 1976a) and approximately 87 % of circulating hydrallazine is bound to plasma proteins (Lesser et al., 1974).

Hydrallazine and its metabolites are rapidly excreted by the kidney and 80 % of an oral dose appears in the urine within 48 hours (Lesser et al., 1974.) The elimination rate of hydrallazine from the plasma does not show a clear cut difference between rapid and slow acetylators of the drug, although it tends to be more prolonged in slow acetylators. In patients with normal renal function, the plasma half-life is 1.7 to 3.0 hours. However, in the presence of chronic renal failure, the plasma half-life is markedly prolonged (7 to 16 hours) [Talseth, 1976b]. Initially, the antihypertensive action of hydrallazine correlates well with plasma concentrations (Zacest and Koch-

Weser, 1972), but, the half-life of the antihypertensive effect is much longer than the plasma half-life (O'Malley et al., 1975a). This may be partly explained by the fact that hydrallazine has been shown to have a special affinity for the walls of muscular arteries and the drug persists much longer in these sites than in the plasma (Moore-Jones and Perry, 1966; Wagner, 1973; Perry et al., 1972).

Following oral ingestion, part of the administered dose is metabolised before reaching the systemic circulation, as biotransformation occurs by the action of N-acetyltransferase within the mucosa of the gastrointestinal tract and as it passes through the liver in the portal circulation (Talseth, 1976c; Reidenberg et al., 1973). This first-pass effect constitutes a major pathway of biodegradation of hydrallazine (Koch-Weser, 1976a). Genetically determined differences in the activity of this enzymatic pathway exist. 'Rapid acetylators' exhibit enhanced activity of this enzymatic pathway and metabolise hydrallazine much more rapidly than 'slow acetylators' (Evans and White, 1964). This difference in enzymatic activity of hepatic and gut N-acetyltransferase is of major clinical importance. For the same administered dose, slow acetylators achieve higher plasma levels (Talseth, 1976a) and therefore exhibit a greater blood pressure lowering effect.

The first-pass effect does not occur following parenteral administration and higher plasma levels are achieved with the same dose given intravenously than when it is ingested (Reidenberg et al., 1973).

3.1.3 Clinical Use

Treatment with hydrallazine is usually initiated with 25mg 2 to 4 times daily, and the dosage may be increased every 2 to 3 days if necessary, until adequate blood pressure control is obtained. The total daily dosage should not exceed 300mg, however, because of the increased risk of hydrallazine induced disseminated lupus-like syndrome (Koch-Weser, 1976a).

The combination of hydrallazine with a diuretic and a β-blocking agent such as propranolol has proved particularly effective (Zacest et al., 1972). β-Blockade reduces the sympathetic mediated reflex increase in cardiac output and therefore alleviates many of the side effects of hydrallazine, and also potentiates its antihypertensive action (Hansson et al., 1971). Other sympathetic blocking agents such as methyldopa, clonidine, guanethidine and reserpine also antagonise the reflex tachycardia of hydrallazine, and in many instances may be substituted for the β-blocking agent with satisfactory results.

Although hydrallazine has traditionally been given four times daily, it has been demonstrated that administration of the same dose in two divided doses provides equally effective blood pressure control (O'Malley et al., 1975a).

3.1.4 Side Effects

Many of the undesirable effects of hydrallazine are due to vasodilatation and the reflex haemodynamic changes which occur; they include tachycardia, palpitation, headache, flushing, nasal congestion, and the precipitation of myocardial ischaemia or congestive heart failure. However, these untoward reactions can often be attenuated or minimised by the co-administration of a β-blocking agent and a diuretic. Even patients with severe underlying coronary disease and limited cardiac reserve can often be managed satisfactorily with this combination.

The chronic administration of hydrallazine can lead to a syndrome resembling the acute rheumatoid state or, when fully developed, disseminated lupus erythematosus. The incidence of this form of hydrallazine toxicity approaches 10 to 20 % in individuals treated with 400mg per day or more; with doses under 200mg daily it has only rarely been reported in some series (Perry, 1973), but has occurred at doses of 100mg daily in others (Standberg et al., 1976). The syndrome is almost always associated with circulating antinuclear antibodies and is more common in Caucasians and slow acetylators of the drug (Perry et al., 1970). This may be due both to the higher and more prolonged plasma levels that are achieved in slow acetylators and the fact that such individuals appear to have a predisposition to the development of lupus (Alarcon-Segovia, 1976). The syndrome is completely reversible upon discontinuance of the drug. However, the antinuclear antibody may persist for 10 years or longer (Perry, 1973).

3.2 Minoxidil

3.2.1 Mode of Action
Minoxidil is a powerful vasodilator which is being investigated but is not yet commercially available. It is a piperidinopyrimidine derivative and is unrelated chemically to the other vasodilating agents. Its pharmacological action is similar to that of hydrallazine and diazoxide in that it exerts a direct relaxant effect on arteriolar smooth muscle (Chidsey et al., 1973).

Minoxidil has little or no effect on the venous capacitance vessels. The decrease in arterial pressure is associated with a fall in peripheral resistance and a reflex increase in cardiac output (O'Malley et al., 1976). Minoxidil produces hyperreninaemia (O'Malley et al., 1975b) and is associated with marked sodium and fluid retention which, if uncontrolled, can lead to massive oedema and congestive heart failure.

3.2.2 Pharmacokinetics
Following absorption, minoxidil rapidly disappears from the plasma (half-life, 2 to 3 hours) and is extensively metabolised (Gottlieb et al., 1971). Its antihypertensive action persists for over 24 hours and appears to bear little relationship to plasma concentrations. Minoxidil accumulates in arterial walls and this may explain its prolonged therapeutic action (Chidsey et al., 1973).

Over 90 % of an oral dose is excreted in the urine within 48 hours, largely in the form of metabolites. Pharmacokinetic data suggest, however, that the elimination of minoxidil depends primarily on metabolic degradation. The total body clearance of the drug is unrelated to the glomerular filtration rate, and excessive accumulation does not occur in the presence of azotemia (Gottlieb et al., 1971).

3.2.3 Clinical Use

Minoxidil is the most potent of the vasodilators and its major indication is control of hypertension which may be life threatening and which has proved resistant to conventional agents. It is especially effective in managing severe hypertension in patients with renal failure and has practically eliminated the need for bilateral nephrectomy for control of hypertension in this situation (Pettinger and Mitchel, 1973).

The usual daily maintenance dose of minoxidil is 10 to 40mg, which can be administered as a single daily dose. Minoxidil should be used in combination with a sympathetic inhibiting agent (usually a β-blocker) and an oral diuretic to counteract the reflex increase in cardiac output and fluid retention which it causes (Gottlieb et al., 1972).

3.2.4 Side Effects

The untoward effects produced by minoxidil are largely those of facial hirsutism and fluid retention. The facial hair growth is particularly distressing in women and can have significant psychological implications. Potentially more serious are pericardial effusions, particularly in patients on haemodialysis (Marquez-Julio and Uldall, 1977), and the peculiar haemorrhagic degenerative lesions which have occurred in the right atrium of dogs. The significance of this lesion is unclear; it has only been observed in dogs treated with very high doses (DuCharme et al., 1973). In our experience, the benefit to risk ratio of the drug seems acceptable for the patient with resistant hypertension.

Pulmonary hypertension can occur during minoxidil therapy related to either a reflex hyperkinetic state or to diminished cardiac efficiency secondary to marked fluid retention (Tarazi et al., 1977a); this latter type, 'congestive pulmonary hypertension', is associated with marked increase in pulmonary wedge pressure and expansion of total blood volume. In contrast, the 'hyperkinetic pulmonary hypertension' is characterised by marked increase in cardiac output, less pronounced rise in pulmonary arterial pressure and smaller expansion in blood volume. Exact characterisation of the pulmonary hypertension will allow a rational decision (more adequate volume depletion versus more effective β-blockade) in the adjustment of therapy (Tarazi et al., 1977b).

3.3 Diazoxide

Diazoxide is a benzothiadiazine derivative closely related chemically to the thiazide diuretics. However, it is a potent vasodilating agent which is devoid of natriuretic activity and in fact causes sodium and fluid retention. In most countries, it is available only for intravenous administration and is used predominantly for the treatment of hypertensive emergencies. The following discussion will be limited to its use in this situation.

3.3.1 Mode of Action

The antihypertensive action of diazoxide is mediated by a reduction of peripheral vascular resistance, presumably by a direct effect on arteriolar smooth muscle (Rubin et al., 1962; Wilson and Okun, 1963). The mechanism by which this occurs is not well understood; however, it may involve antagonism of the smooth muscle action of calcium (Janis and Triggle, 1973).

As with hydrallazine and minoxidil, the antihypertensive effect of diazoxide is associated with a sympathetically mediated increase in heart rate and cardiac output, which partially counteracts its antihypertensive action (Hamby et al., 1968; Koch-Weser, 1976b). Renal blood flow and glomerular filtration rate may fall transiently immediately following administration, but these return to pretreatment levels within a few hours (Hamby et al., 1968; Johnson, 1971; Lockwood et al., 1963). Diazoxide has little effect on venous capacitance vessels (Thirwell and Zsoter, 1972) and no direct action on the myocardium (Koch-Weser, 1974).

3.3.2 Clinical Use

In many instances, diazoxide is an effective agent for the management of hypertensive emergencies. It is particularly effective in situations where prompt reduction of blood pressure is desirable, such as hypertensive encephalopathy, malignant hypertension and eclampsia. It should be administered as a *rapid* intravenous injection (Mroczek et al., 1971) of 300mg in adults or approximately 5mg/kg in children. Diazoxide is highly protein bound and the entire dose must be given rapidly (within 15 to 20 seconds) so that high initial concentrations of free drug are attained, otherwise binding by plasma proteins will neutralise its effects (Sellers and Koch-Weser, 1969). Its maximum antihypertensive effect occurs within 5 minutes and the blood pressure is promptly reduced, usually to normotensive levels in 75 to 85% of patients (Miller et al., 1969). The antihypertensive effect of a single dose usually persists for 6 to 18 hours or longer. The concomitant administration of intravenous frusemide will prevent fluid retention and may enhance and prolong its therapeutic effect. Hypotension occurs uncommonly and is generally transient and of little clinical consequence.

Diazoxide is relatively contraindicated in patients with coronary and cerebral vascular insufficiency in whom a rapid reduction in pressure could precipitate coronary (Kanada et al., 1976) or cerebral ischaemia. However, it has recently been shown that arterial pressure can often be gradually reduced in such patients without undue risk, by intermittently injecting smaller doses of diazoxide (50 to 100mg intravenously) at approximately 15 minute intervals until adequate blood pressure control is achieved (Wilson and Vidt, 1978). Because it increases cardiac output and the left ventricular ejection velocity, diazoxide is unsuitable for managing hypertension associated with dissecting aortic aneurysm.

Although diazoxide causes the abrupt cessation of labour when used in the treatment of toxaemia, this effect is readily overcome with the use of oxytoxic drugs (Landesman et al., 1968). Diazoxide can also cause significant hyperglycaemia, especially in diabetics, and the blood glucose should be determined daily while it is being used.

3.4 Sodium Nitroprusside

Sodium nitroprusside is a powerful vasodilating agent and is the most consistently effective drug available for the management of hypertensive crises (Gifford, 1977). Its antihypertensive potency is unequalled by any other agent and it is universally effective in the treatment of hypertensive emergencies, regardless of aetiology.

3.4.1 Mode of Action
The antihypertensive action of sodium nitroprusside results from a direct effect of the nitroso group on vascular smooth muscle, causing vasodilatation of both the arterioles and venules (Shah, 1977). Although it causes an increase in heart rate, it differs from the other vasodilators in that it does not incite a reflex increase in cardiac output. This is probably due to a relaxant effect on venous capacitance vessels resulting in a reduction of venous return to the heart (Tarazi et al., 1977). Because it reduces both cardiac preload and afterload, it improves left ventricular performance in patients with refractory heart failure, even when hypertension is minimal or absent (Palmer and Lasseter, 1975).

3.4.2 Clinical Use
Because its antihypertensive action lasts for less than 1 to 2 minutes, sodium nitroprusside must be administered by continuous intravenous infusion. One of the disadvantages of sodium nitroprusside is that the infusion requires constant monitoring by experienced personnel within the confines of an intensive care unit. The infusion is usually begun, with a solution containing 100mg/litre, at a rate of 20 micro drops per minute. The blood pressure begins to fall within 30 seconds and care must be taken to prevent hypotension; however, with expert titration, the blood pressure can be maintained at any desired level. Because its action is so evanescent, the pressure quickly rises to hypertensive levels within 2 to 3 minutes of the infusion being discontinued.

Although effective in virtually every form of hypertensive crisis, sodium nitroprusside is the drug of choice for hypertension associated with acute myocardial infarction and left ventricular failure, because of its favourable effect on cardiac performance (Chaterjee et al., 1973; Miller et al., 1975). It is also safer than diazoxide in the management of hypertension associated with acute coronary insufficiency, cerebrovascular insufficiency and intracranial haemorrhage, where careful blood pressure regulation is required and prolonged hypotension might be detrimental (Gifford, 1975).

3.4.3 Side Effects

The untoward effects produced by sodium nitroprusside include sweating, muscular twitching, nausea, anxiety, and apprehension, which are generally manifestations of rapid reduction in blood pressure and are promptly relieved by decreasing the infusion rate or stopping it temporarily.

Nitroprusside is metabolised to cyanogen, largely by erythrocytes, and is converted to thiocyanate by the liver and excreted by the kidney. Occasionally, with prolonged administration (usually more than 3 days), acute thiocyanate intoxication may result as manifested by delirium and psychosis. This is more common in the presence of renal insufficiency where thiocyanate excretion is reduced. If sodium nitroprusside is administered for longer than 72 hours, daily serum thiocyanate determinations should be obtained and therapy should be withdrawn whenever the concentration exceeds 12mg/100ml.

4. Angiotensin II Analogues and Converting Enzyme Inhibitors

There are several compounds at present under investigation which specifically inhibit the pharmacological effect of angiotensin II. Synthetic analogues such as saralasin (P-113; sar[1]-ala[8]-angiotensin II) compete with circulating angiotensin II for receptor sites within vascular smooth muscle and the adrenal cortex (Streeten et al., 1977). The converting enzyme inhibitors, such as compound SQ-20881, inhibit the enzymatic conversion of inactive angiotensin I to the potent vasoconstrictor substance, angiotensin II (Streeten et al., 1977).

At present, these agents are important research tools for investigating the participation of the renin-angiotensin system in various forms of hypertension (Case et al., 1976, 1977). Because they are useful in identifying hypertension that is angiotensin dependent, they may prove valuable in the future selection of patients with renovascular hypertension who will benefit from surgical treatment (Streeten et al., 1975). They may also prove useful in the management of hypertensive crises associated with high circulating levels of angiotensin II (Gavras et al., 1974); however, these agents must be administered parenterally, and at present they are of no use in the chronic treatment of hypertension.

More recently Ondetti et al. (1977) have developed an orally active converting enzyme inhibitor (SQ14225). Early experience with this compound has been promising (Cody et al., 1978a; Gavras et al., 1978); patients with either essential or renovascular hypertension resistant to other antihypertensive agents have responded to SQ14225 either alone or in association with a low sodium diet (10mEq/day) or

Table IV. Steps in the medical treatment of hypertension

Step 1:
Oral Diuretic (usually thiazide or related diuretic; use frusemide if azotaemia present)

Step 2:
Add a sympathetic depressant:
a) β-Blocker (e.g. propranolol, 40mg bid-120mg qid or 240mg bid); *or*
b) Methyldopa (250mg bid-500mg qid); *or*
c) Clonidine (0.075-0.1mg bid-0.6mg qid); *or*
d) Reserpine (0.25mg qd); or
c) Labetalol (100-200mg tid or qid)

Step 3:
Add a vasodilator:
a) Hydrallazine (25mg bid-75mg qid); *or*
b) Prazosin[1] (small initial dose, then 2mg bid-10mg bid)

Step 4:
Add a more potent sympathetic depressant:
Guanethidine[2] (10-100mg qd or more)

---

1   It may be possible to use prazosin as an alternative in step 2 instead of one of the sympathetic depressant drugs.
N.B. First dose of prazosin must be low and preferably given at bedtime.
2   Other adrenergic neurone blocking drugs (e.g. bethanidine, debrisoquine) may be used as an alternative to guanethidine.

---

diuretic therapy. In our experience, basal plasma renin activity was not a good predictor of blood pressure responsiveness. The exact mechanism by which arterial pressure is lowered is still not clear; interference with production of angiotensin II is undoubtedly important but increase in bradykinin or other yet unspecified drug effects may play a role. The reduction in blood pressure is related to lowering of TPR; cardiac output and heart rate are not significantly altered (Cody et al., 1978b). Haemodynamic responses to upright posture were not interfered with by the converting enzyme inhibitor even when associated with sodium depletion or diuretic therapy, indicating that baroceptor reflexes were effectively operative.

Side effects of SQ14225 included fever and a morbilliform rash that developed with doses exceeding 600mg/day; this may be associated with rhonchi and some proteinuria. The syndrome appears to be dose dependent and disappears within 48 hours of discontinuing the drug. Transient mild to moderate itching has developed in some patients; it is often unobtrusive and usually easily tolerated. Rapid reduction of blood pressure, particularly if SQ14225 is associated with sodium depletion, can be accompanied by a rise in serum creatinine and BUN.

Table V. Contraindications and side effects of antihypertensive agents

Drug	Side effects		Contraindications[2]
	Innocuous, but sometimes annoying	Harmful or potentially harmful	
Oral diuretics a) Thiazide type	Dry mouth Unpleasant taste Weakness Muscle cramps Hyperuricaemia (sometimes with gout) Gastrointestinal disturbances	Hypokalaemia Hyponatraemia[1] Hyperglycaemia Hypercalcaemia[1] Azotaemia[1] Skin rash[1] Photosensitivity[1] Purpura[1] Marrow depression[1] Lithium toxicity[1] (pts on lithium therapy)	Persistent anuria/oliguria Advanced renal failure Hyponatraemia
b) Spirono- lactone	Drowsiness Hirsutism Menstrual irregularities Gynaecomastia Dry mouth Unpleasant taste Gastrointestinal disturbances	Hyperkalaemia[1] Hyponatraemia[1]	Renal failure Hyperkalaemia Hyponatraemia
Reserpine	Bradycardia Lethargy Lassitude Impotence Diarrhoea Nasal congestion	Depression[1] Activation of peptic ulcer[1] Parkinsonian state[1]	Depression (past or present) Active peptic ulcer Parkinsonism
Methyldopa	Drowsiness Lethargy Dry mouth Impotence + Direct Coombs' test Nasal congestion	Abnormal liver function tests Hepatitis[1] Drug fever[1] Haemolytic anaemia[1] Retroperitoneal fibrosis[1] Skin rash[1] Orthostatic hypotension Depression[1]	Coombs' positive haemolytic anaemia Hepatic disease

Table V. (continued)

Drug	Side effects		Contraindications[2]
	Innocuous, but sometimes annoying	Harmful or potentially harmful	
Guanethidine	Bradycardia Exercise hypotension Diarrhoea (especially following meals) Weakness Retrograde ejaculation or impotence Nasal congestion	Orthostatic hypotension (potentially harmful in patients with cerebral or myocardial ischaemia and advanced renal insufficiency) Drug sensitivity (rare)[1]	Interacts with tricyclic antidepressants, sympathomimetic amines
Propranolol[3]	Bradycardia Weakness Lethargy Gastrointestinal disturbances	Congestive heart failure (only in pts with diminished cardiac reserve) Bronchospasm[1] (in patients with asthmatic propensity) Hypoglycaemia[1] (propranolol can mask the warning symptoms in insulin dependent diabetics) Aggravation of arterial insufficiency[1] (in pts with peripheral occlusive arterial disease) Nightmares[1] Insomnia[1] Hallucinations[1] Depression[1] Hyperglycaemia Hyperosmolar coma[1] Abnormal liver function tests[1] (rare) Allergic reactions[1] (rare) Leucopenia[1] (rare) Thrombocytopenia[1] (rare)	Bronchial asthma Second or third degree heart block Congestive heart failure (unless due to an arrhythmia amenable to therapy with propranolol or uncontrolled hypertension) 'Brittle' diabetes mellitus
Clonidine	Dry mouth Drowsiness Lethargy Impotence Gastrointestinal disturbances Constipation	'Rebound hypertension' when abruptly discontinued Parotid pain[1] (rare)	None[2]

Table V. (continued)

Drug	Side effects		Contraindications[2]
	Innocuous, but sometimes annoying	Harmful or potentially harmful	
Hydrallazine	Tachycardia[4] Palpitation[4] Headache[4] Flushing[4] Nasal congestion Gastrointestinal disturbances	Aggravation of angina[1,4] Precipitation of congestive failure in patients with myocardial disease[1] Lupus-like syndrome[1] Drug fever[1] Skin rash[1] Psychosis[1] Marrow suppression[1]	Symptomatic arteriosclerotic heart disease (unless used with propranolol)
Prazosin	Headache Palpitation Drowsiness Dizziness Nausea	Sudden collapse and loss of consciousness (usually after initial dose; minimise by always using low first dose)	None[2]

1   Usually requires cessation of therapy, at least temporarily.
2   Hypersensitivity is obviously a contraindication to any drug and will not be repeated for each.
3   Some of these side effects are modified or absent with other β-blocking agents due to differences in pharmacological properties (CNS effects and aggravation of arterial insufficiency are more common with propranolol than with other β-blockers).
4   These side effects are often minimised or prevented by the co-administration of a β-blocker.

In summary, the indications are that this new compound may be a useful addition to our therapeutic armamentarium. Like other antihypertensives, it frequently needs to be associated with effective diuretic therapy. Its use is still restricted to investigational studies.

5. Treatment Regimens

A rational approach to therapy based upon a therapeutic regimen which is designed for a specific pathophysiological abnormality is obviously the most desirable approach to the treatment of hypertension. However, the means are rarely available for determining precise mechanisms in individual patients, and treatment is of necessity, largely empirical. The 'stepped care' programme (table IV) has gained wide use and exemplifies the empirical approach to therapy. Although it undoubtedly leads to unnecessary therapy in some instances, it is generally effective in eventually providing adequate blood pressure control.

5.1 Mild Hypertension

In patients with mild hypertension (e.g. diastolic pressure 90 to 115mm Hg), therapy is usually instituted with an oral diuretic of the thiazide variety. In at least 30% of cases, the oral diuretic alone will reduce the blood pressure to normotensive levels ($<$140/90mm Hg). However, if the pressure remains elevated after 4 to 6 weeks of therapy, a sympathetic depressant should be added (step 2, table IV). The choice of a sympatholytic agent for step 2 depends more on side effects and the presence of contraindications to certain drugs (see tables V and VI) than on efficacy, because when employed in combination with therapeutic doses of a diuretic, they are approximately equal in regard to therapeutic potency. β-Blockers are usually well tolerated by most patients; however, methyldopa, clonidine or reserpine, and possibly labetalol, are suitable substitutes. Reserpine seems to be tolerated least by the majority of patients, although it has the advantage of being relatively inexpensive and long acting, requiring only one dose daily.

When the hypertension does not respond to the combination of a diuretic and sympathetic blocking agent, a vasodilator such as hydrallazine can be added to the regimen as step 3. The co-administration of hydrallazine with a β-blocker prevents the reflex tachycardia and increase in cardiac output caused by hydrallazine. To a lesser degree, methyldopa, clonidine and reserpine also blunt the reflex tachycardia of hydrallazine and thus enhance its therapeutic effect; thus, hydrallazine can be used in step 3 regardless of the sympatholytic agent employed in step 2. Whether or not prazosin in practice is a suitable substitute for hydrallazine is not known at present. However, because prazosin does not usually cause reflex tachycardia and an increase in cardiac output, presumably it could be used in place of the sympatholytic agents in step 2, in which case a sympathetic inhibitor could later be added to the regimen if necessary. A β-blocker may be helpful in this instance as the sympathetic blockade produced would then include both α- and β-adrenoceptors.

5.2 Moderate to Severe Hypertension

The higher the pretreatment blood pressure, the less likely an oral diuretic agent alone will be effective in controlling the blood pressure. Consequently, when the diastolic pressure is greater than 115mm Hg, it is generally advisable to institute therapy with an oral diuretic and a sympathetic depressant agent simultaneously (step 1 and 2). When the pretreatment diastolic pressure is greater than 130mm Hg, treatment should be initiated with all three classes of agents simultaneously (steps 1, 2 and 3).

Table VI. Special indications and contraindications for certain antihypertensive drugs

Symptoms or conditions	Drugs which may be beneficial	Drugs which may aggravate the condition
Headache	Methyldopa Reserpine Propranolol[1] Clonidine	Hydrallazine Prazosin
Constipation	Guanethidine Reserpine	Ganglion blocking agents Clonidine
Chronic diarrhoea	Clonidine Ganglion blocking agents	Guanethidine Reserpine
Depression	Pargyline	Reserpine
Palpitations and heart consciousness (cardiac neurosis)	Guanethidine Reserpine Propranolol[2]	Hydrallazine Prazosin
Anxiety-tension state and/or insomnia	Methyldopa Reserpine Clonidine	Pargyline
Essential tremor	Propranolol[1]	—
Postural dizziness	—	Ganglion blocking agents Guanethidine Pargyline
Hepatic dysfunction	—	Methyldopa Pargyline
Gout	—	Thiazide and 'loop' diuretics

1   The efficacy of the other β-blocking agents has not been established in these situations.
2   Other β-blocking agents are suitable alternatives to propranolol in this situation.

Table VII. Special indications and contraindications for some antipressor drugs in complicated hypertension

Complication	Preferred drugs	Drugs to avoid or to use with extreme caution
Congestive heart failure	Diuretics Methyldopa Guanethidine Clonidine Prazosin	β-Blocking agents (unless patient receiving digitalis and diuretic)
Azotaemia	Methyldopa Hydrallazine Propranolol[1] Frusemide Clonidine Reserpine Prazosin	Oral diuretics (except frusemide) Guanethidine
Cerebrovascular insufficiency	Oral diuretics Methyldopa Hydrallazine Propranolol[1] Clonidine Prazosin	Guanethidine
Coronary insufficiency	Oral diuretics Propranolol[1] Methyldopa Clonidine Reserpine	Hydrallazine Guanethidine

1   Other β-blocking agents may be used in place of propranolol.

5.3 Resistant Hypertension

If the blood pressure is not adequately controlled by a combined diuretic/sympatholytic/vasodilator regimen, the clinician should stop and re-investigate the patient for possible underlying factors which may be contributing to the lack of effective blood pressure control. If the patient has adhered strictly to his drug regimen, he has effectively demonstrated resistance to conventional drug therapy. Possible causes, lines of investigations and therapeutic approaches have recently been discussed (Gifford and Tarazi, 1978). Patients in this category constitute a relatively small group in whom the positive yield of such an evaluation is correspondingly greater. The economic aspects of such an undertaking are therefore less formidable and more justifiable.

Assuming that non-compliance, 'pseudotolerance' due to plasma volume expansion, unfavourable drug interactions and secondary forms of hypertension have been excluded as possible causes of drug resistance, an adrenergic neurone blocking drug such as guanethidine can be added to the other agents as step 4. Because of the high incidence of side effects, however, guanethidine should be reserved for the treatment of severe hypertension which has not responded to combination therapy with adequate doses of a diuretic, sympatholytic agent and a vasodilator (steps 1, 2 and 3).

When a β-blocker such as propranolol is used in step 2, it is sometimes helpful to use the α-adrenoceptor blocker phenoxybenzamine in step 4 rather than guanethidine. Orthostatic hypotension is sometimes a major problem when either guanethidine or phenoxybenzamine is combined with propranolol, and it is often advisable to reduce the dose of propranolol before adding either one of these agents. Theoretically, prazosin, because of its α-adrenoceptor blocking effect, could be used in step 4 in place of phenoxybenzamine (if it has not already been used in step 3); however, we are not sure of the therapeutic efficacy of this combination.

In the small number of patients who continue to remain resistant to therapy, consideration should be given to the use of minoxidil. In this situation, minoxidil can be substituted for the vasodilating agent used in step 3 or simply added to the other antihypertensive agents.

5.4 Hypertensive Emergencies and Presence of Complications

In the event of a hypertensive emergency, such as hypertensive encephalopathy, congestive heart failure, coronary insufficiency or intracranial haemorrhage, a parenteral agent should be given to control the blood pressure until the oral regimen becomes effective. When cardiovascular or renal complications are already present, the regimen may have to be modified to avoid certain drugs which might worsen the clinical situation (table VII).

Acknowledgement

We thank Mrs Aldona Raulinaitis, Mrs Elizabeth Libby, Mrs Marge Cook, Mrs Veronica Hiebel and Mrs Jean Wollam for their skillful assistance.

References

Abboud, F.M.: Effects of sodium, angiotensin and steroids on vascular reactivity in man. Federation Proceedings 33: 144-149 (1974).

Abboud, F.M.; Eckstein, J.W. and Wendling, M.G.: Early potentiation of the vasoconstrictor action of norepinephrine by guanethidine. Proceedings of the Society for Experimental Biology and Medicine 110: 489-492 (1962).

Ablad, B. and Johnsson, G.: Comparative effects of intra-arterially administered hydralazine and sodium nitrite on blood flow and volume of forearm. Acta Pharmacologica et Toxicologica 20: 1-15 (1963).

Alarcon-Segovia, D.: Drug-induced antinuclear antibodies and lupus syndromes. Drugs 12: 69-77 (1976).

Alper, J.H.; Flacke, W. and Krayer, O.: Pharmacology of reserpine and its implications for anesthesia. Anesthesiology 24: 524-542 (1963).

Altura, B.M.: Pharmacological effects of alpha-methyldopa, alpha-methylnorepinephrine, and octopamine on rat arteriolar, arterial and terminal vascular smooth muscle. Circulation Research 36 & 37 (Suppl. 1): 233-240 (1975).

Amery, A. and Deloof, W.: Cheese reaction during debrisoquine treatment. Lancet 2: 613 (1970).

Anavekar, S.N.; Louis, W.J.; Morgan, T.P.; Doyle, A.E. and Johnston, C.I.: The relationship of plasma levels of pindolol in hypertensive patients to effects on blood pressure, plasma renin and plasma noradrenaline levels. Clinical and Experimental Pharmacology and Physiology 2: 203-212 (1975).

Anderson, C.C. and Gabriel, R.: Poor hypotensive response and tachyphylaxis following intravenous labetalol. Current Medical Research and Opinion 5: 424 (1978).

Anderson, J.; Godfrey, B.E.; Hill, D.M.; Munro-Faure, A.D. and Sheldon, J.: A comparison of the effects of hydrochlorothiazide and of frusemide in the treatment of hypertensive patients. Quarterly Journal of Medicine, New Series 40: 541-560 (1971).

Anderson, K.V.; Brettell, H.R. and Aikawa, J.K.: C^{14}-labelled hydrochlorothiazide in human beings. Archives of Internal Medicine 107: 168-174 (1961).

Armstrong, B.; Stevens, N. and Doll, R.: Retrospective study of the association between use of Rauwolfia derivatives and breast cancer in English women. Lancet 2: 672-675 (1974).

Au, W.Y.W.; Dring, L.G.; Grahame-Smith, D.G.; Isaac, P. and Williams, R.T.: The metabolism of ^{14}C-labelled α-methyldopa in normal and hypertensive human subjects. Biochemical Journal 129: 1-10 (1972).

Aviado, D.M.: Hemodynamic effects of ganglion blocking drugs. Circulation Research 8: 304-314 (1960).

Aviado, D.M.: Treatment of essential hypertension; in Krantz and Carr (Eds) Pharmacologic Principles of Medical Practice, pp. 535-555 (Wilkins and Williams, Baltimore 1972).

Awan, N.A.; Miller, R.R. and Mason, D.T.: Comparison of effects of nitroprusside and prazosin on left ventricular function and the peripheral circulation in chronic refractory congestive heart failure. Circulation 57: 152-159 (1978).

Awan, N.A.; Miller, R.R.; Maxwell, K. and Mason D.T.: Effects of prazosin on forearm resistance and capacitance vessels. Clinical Pharmacology and Therapeutics 22: 79-84 (1977).

Ayitey-Smith, E. and Varma, D.R.: Mechanism of the hypotensive action of methyldopa in normal and immunosympathectomized rats. British Journal of Pharmacology 40: 186-193 (1970).

Baba, W.I.; Tudhope, G.R. and Wilson, G.M.: Triamterene, a new diuretic drug. I. Studies in normal men and in adrenalectomized rats. British Medical Journal 3: 756-760 (1962).

Baer, J.E.; Leidy, L.; Brooks, A.V. and Beyer, K.H.: The physiological disposition of chlorothiazide (diuril) in the dog. Journal of Pharmacology and Experimental Therapeutics 125: 295-302 (1959).

Bailey, R.R. and Neale, T.J.: Rapid clonidine withdrawal with blood pressure overshoot exaggerated by beta-blockade. British Medical Journal 1: 942-943 (1976).

Baum, T.; Shropshire, A.T. and Varner, L.L.: Contribution of the central nervous system to the action of several antihypertensive agents (methyldopa, hydralazine and guanethidine). Journal of Pharmacology and Experimental Therapeutics 182: 135-144 (1972).

Beermann, B.; Dalen, E. and Lindstrom, B.: Elimination of furosemide in healthy subjects and in those with renal failure. Clinical Pharmacology and Therapeutics 22: 70-78 (1977).

Beermann, B.; Groschinsky-Grind, M. and Rosen, A.: Absorption, metabolism, and excretion of hydrochlorothiazide. Clinical Pharmacology and Therapeutics 19: 531-537 (1976).

Beermann, B.; Hellstrom, K.; Lindstrom, B. and Rosen, A.: Binding-site interaction of chlorthalidone and acetazolamide, two drugs transported by red blood cells. Clinical Pharmacology and Therapeutics 17: 424-432 (1975).

Beisenherz, G.; Koss, F.W.; Klatt, L. and Binder, B.: Distribution of radioactivity in the tissues and excretory products of rats and rabbits following administration of C^{14}-hygroton®. Archives Internationales de Pharmacodynamie et de Therapie 161: 76-93 (1966).

Bengtsson, C.; Johnsson, G. and Regardh, C.G.: Plasma levels and effects of metoprolol on blood pressure and heart rate in hypertensive patients after an acute dose and between two doses during long-term treatment. Clinical Pharmacology and Therapeutics 17: 400-408 (1974).

Beumer, H.M.: Adverse effects of beta-adrenergic receptor blocking drugs on respiratory function. Drugs 7: 130-138 (1974).

Beyer, K.H.: The mechanism of action of chlorothiazide. Annals of New York Academy of Sciences 71: 363-379 (1958).

Beyer, K.H. and Baer, J.E.: The site and mode of action of some sulfonamide-derived diuretics. Medical Clinics of North America 59: 735-750 (1975).

Beyer, K.H.; Baer, J.E.; Michaelson, J.K. and Russo, H.F.: Renotropic characteristics of ethacrynic acid: a phenoxyacetic saluretic-diuretic agent. Journal of Pharmacology and Experimental Therapeutics 147: 1-22 (1965).

Bhatia, S.K. and Frohlich, E.D.: Hemodynamic comparison of agents useful in hypertensive emergencies. American Heart Journal 85: 367-373 (1973).

Bianchetti, G.; Graziani, G.; Brancaccio, D.; Morganti, A.; Leonetti, G.; Manfrin, M.; Sega, R.; Gomeni, R.; Ponticelli, C. and Morselli, P.L.: Pharmacokinetics and effects of propranolol in terminal uraemic patients and in patients undergoing regular dialysis treatment. Clinical Pharmacokinetics 1: 373-384 (1976).

Blum, I.; Doron, M.; Laron, Z.; Atsmon, A. and Tiqva, P.: Prevention of hypoglycemic attacks by propranolol in a patient suffering from insulinoma. Diabetes 24: 535-537 (1975).

Bock, K.D.; Merguet, P. and Heimsoth, V.K.: Effect of clonidine on regional blood flow and its use in the treatment of hypertension; in Onesti, Kim and Moyer (Eds) Hypertension: Mechanisms and Management, p.395 (Grune and Stratton, New York 1973).

Bolli, P.; Waal-Manning, H.J.; Wood, A.J. and Simpson, F.O.: Experience with labetalol in hypertension. British Journal of Clinical Pharmacology 3 (Suppl. 3): 765-771 (1976).

Bolli, P.; Wood, A.J.; Phelan, E.L.; Lee, D.R. and Simpson, F.O.: Prazosin: Preliminary clinical and pharmacological observations. Clinical Science and Molecular Medicine 48: 177s-179s (1975).

Bolzano, K.: Prazosin, a new quinazoline derivate in the treatment of essential hypertension; in Cotton (Ed) Proceedings of a Symposium held at the Centre Interprofessionnel, Geneva, 8 March 1974, pp.144-148 (Elsevier, New York 1974).

Boura, A.L.A. and Green, A.F.: Adrenergic neurone blocking agents. Annual Review of Pharmacology 5: 183-212 (1965).

Braunwald, E.; Chidsey, C.A.; Harrison, D.C.; Gaffney, T.E. and Kahler, R.L.: Studies on the function of the adrenergic nerve endings in the heart. Circulation 28: 958-969 (1963).

Bravo, E.L.; Tarazi, R.C. and Dustan, H.P.: On the mechanism of suppressed plasma renin activity during beta-adrenergic blockade with propranolol. Journal of Laboratory and Clinical Medicine 83: 119-128 (1974).

Bravo, E.L.; Tarazi, R.C. and Dustan, H.P.: Beta-adrenergic blockade in diuretic-treated patients with essential hypertension. New England Journal of Medicine 292: 66-70 (1975a).

Bravo, E.L.; Tarazi, R.C.; Dustan, H.P. and Lewis, J.W.: Dissociation between renin and arterial pressure responses to beta-adrenergic blockade in human essential hypertension. Circulation Research 36 & 36 (Suppl.1): 241-247 (1975b).

Brettell, H.R.; Aikawa, J.K. and Gordon, G.S.: Studies with chlorothiazide tagged with radioactive carbon (C^{14}) in human beings. Archives of Internal Medicine 106: 109-115 (1960).

Brettell, H.R.; Smith, J.G. and Aikawa, J.K.: S^{35}-labeled bendroflumethiazide in human beings. Archives of Internal Medicine 113: 373-377 (1964).

Briant, R.H.; Dollery, C.T.; Fenyvesi, T. and George, C.F.: Assessment of selective beta-adrenoceptor blockade in man. British Journal of Pharmacology 49: 106-114 (1973).

Briant, R.H.; Reid, J.L. and Dollery, C.T.: Interaction between clonidine and desipramine in man. British Medical Journal 1: 522-523 (1973).

Brogden, R.N.; Heel, R.C.; Speight, T.M. and Avery, G.S.: Prazosin: A review of its pharmacological properties and therapeutic efficacy in hypertension. Drugs 14: 163-197 (1977).

Brunner, L.; Imhof, P. and Jack, D.: Relation between plasma concentration and cardiovascular effects of oral oxprenolol in man. European Journal of Clinical Pharmacology 8: 3-9 (1975).

Buhler, F.R.; Laragh, J.H.; Baer, L.; Vaughan, E.D. and Brunner, H.R.: Propranolol inhibition of renin-secretion. A specific approach to diagnosis and treatment of renin-dependent hypertensive diseases. New England Journal of Medicine 287: 1209-1214 (1972).

Buhs, R.P.; Beck, J.L.; Speth, O.C.; Smith, J.L.; Trenner, N.R.; Cannon, P.J. and Laragh, J.H.: The metabolism of methyldopa in hypertensive human subjects. Journal of Pharmacology and Experimental Therapeutics 143: 205-214 (1964).

Burg, M. and Green, N.: Effect of ethacrynic acid on the thick ascending limb of Henle's loop. Kidney International 4: 301-308 (1973).

Byck, R.: Drugs and the treatment of psychiatric disorders; in Goodman and Gilman (Eds) The Pharmacological Basis of Therapeutics, pp.167-169 (MacMillan, New York 1975).

Calesnick, B.; Christensen, J.A. and Richter, M.: Absorption and excretion of furosemide-S^{35} in human subjects. Proceedings of the Soceity of Experimental Biology and Medicine 123: 17-22 (1966).

Calesnick, B.; Sheppard, H. and Bowen, N.: Direct comparison of C^{14} chlorothiazide and T^3 hydrochlorothiazide in man. Federation Proceedings 20: 409 (1961).

Cambridge, D.; Davey, M.J. and Massingham, R.: The pharmacology of antihypertensive drugs with special reference to vasodilators, α-adrenergic blocking agents and prazosin. Medical Journal of Australia 2 (Special Suppl. 1): 2-7 (1977).

Carlsson, A. and Lindqvist, M.: In vivo decarboxylation of α-methyldopa and α-methyl metatyrosine. Acta Physiologica Scandinavica 54: 87-94 (1962).

Carrier, O., Jr.: in Pharmacology of the Peripheral Autonomic Nervous System, pp.120-123 (Year Book Medical Publishers, Chicago 1972).

Carruthers, S.G.; Kelly, J.G.; McDevitt, D.G.; Shanks, R.G. and Walsh, M.J.: Duration of action of beta-blocking drugs. British Medical Journal 2: 177 (1973).

Carstairs, K.D.; Breckenridge, A.; Dollery, C.T. and Worlledge, S.M.: Incidence of a positive direct Coombs test in patients on α-methyldopa. Lancet 2: 133-135 (1966).

Case, D.B.; Wallace, J.M.; Keim, H.J.; Weber, M.A.; Drayer, J.I.M.; White, R.P.; Sealey, J.E. and Laragh, J.H.: Estimating renin participation in hypertension: Superiority of converting enzyme inhibitor over saralasin. American Journal of Medicine 61: 790-796 (1976).

Case, D.B.; Wallace, J.M.; Keim, H.J.; Weber, M.A.; Sealey, J.E. and Laragh, J.H.: Possible role of renin in hypertension as suggested by renin-sodium profiling and inhibition of converting enzyme. New England Journal of Medicine 296: 641-646 (1977).

Cerasi, E.; Luft, R. and Efendic, S.: Effect of adrenergic blocking agents on insulin response to glucose infusion in man. Acta Endocrinologica 69: 335-346 (1972).

Chamberlain, D.A. and Howard, J.: Guanethidine and methyldopa: A haemodynamic study. British Heart Journal 26: 528-536 (1964).

Chang, C.C.; Costa, E. and Brodie, B.B.: Interaction of guanethidine with adrenergic neurons. Journal of Pharmacology and Experimental Therapeutics 147: 303-312 (1965).

Chaterjee, K.; Parmley, W.W.; Ganz, W.; Forrester, J.; Walinsky, P.; Crexels, C. and Swan, H.J.C.: Hemodynamic and metabolic responses to vasodilator therapy in acute myocardial infarction. Circulation 48: 1183-1193 (1973).

Chidsey, C.A. and Gottlieb, T.B.: The pharmacologic basis of antihypertensive therapy. The role of vasodilator drugs. Progress in Cardiovascular Diseases 17: 99-113 (1974).

Chidsey, C.A.; Braunwald, E. and Morrow, A.G.: Reserpine and noradrenaline stores. Lancet 2: 458-459 (1962).

Chidsey, C.A.; Braunwald, E.; Morrow, A.G. and Mason, D.T.: Myocardial norepinephrine concentration in man. Effects of reserpine and of congestive heart failure. New England Journal of Medicine 269: 653-658 (1963).

Chidsey, C.A.; Gottlieb, T.B.; Pluss, R.G.; Orcutt, J.C. and Weil, J.V.: The use of vasodilators and beta-adrenergic blockade in hypertension; in Onesti, Kim and Moyer (Eds) Hypertension: Mechanisms and Management, pp.357-367 (Grune and Stratton, New York 1973).

Cleaveland, C.R. and Shand, D.G.: Effect of route of administration on the relationship between beta-adrenergic blockade and plasma propranolol level. Clinical Pharmacology and Therapeutics 13: 181-185 (1971).

Cody, R.J.; Tarazi, R.C.; Bravo, E.L. and Fouad, F.M.: Hemodynamics of orally-active converting enzyme inhibitor (SQ 14225) in hypertensive patients. Amer. J. Cardiol. 41: 402 (1978a).

Cody, R.J.; Tarazi, R.C.; Bravo, E.L. and Fouad, F.M.: Haemodynamics of orally-active converting enzyme inhibitor (SQ14225) in hypertensive patients. Clinical Science and Molecular Medicine 55: 453-459 (1978b).

Cohen, A.I.; Hartman, A.D.; Hinsvark, O.N.; Kraus, P.F. and Zazulak, W.: Physiological disposition of a new diuretic, ^{14}C-metolazone, in dogs. Journal of Pharmaceutical Sciences 62: 931-936 (1973).

Cohen, R.A. (Ed): False neurochemical transmitters. Annals of Internal Medicine 65: 347-362 (1966).

Cohen, R.A.; Maxmen, J.S.; Ragheb, M.; Baleiron, H.; Zaleski, E.J. and Bing, R.J.: Effects of alpha-methyldopa on the myocardial blood flow, utilizing the coincidence counting method. Journal of Clinical Pharmacology 7: 77-83 (1967).

Cohn, J.N.; Liptak, T.E. and Freis, E.D.: Hemodynamic effects of guanethidine in man. Circulation Research 12: 298-307 (1963).

Collins, J.S. and Pek, P.: Pharmacokinetics of prazosin, a new antihypertensive compound. Clinical and Experimental Pharmacology and Physiology 2: 445-446 (1975).

Collste, P.; Haglund, K.; Frisk-Holmberg, M.; Orme, M.L.E.; Rawlins, M.D. and Ostman, J.: Pharmacokinetics and pharmacodynamics of alprenolol in the treatment of hypertension. European Journal of Clinical Pharmacology 10: 89-95 (1976).

Conolly, M.E.: Clonidine in the treatment of hypertension; in Davies and Reid (Eds) Central Action of Drugs in Blood Pressure Regulation, pp.268-275 (University Park Press, Baltimore 1975).

Conradi, E.C.; Gaffney, T.E.; Fink, D.A. and Vangrow, J.S.: Reversal of sympathetic nerve blockade: A comparison of dopa, dopamine and norepinephrine with methyl-α-methylated analogues. Journal of Pharmacology and Experimental Therapeutics 150: 26-33 (1965).

Constantine, J.W.; McShane, W.K.; Scriabine, A. and Hess, H.: Analysis of the hypotensive action of prazosin; in Onesti, Kim and Moyer (Eds) Hypertension: Mechanisms and Management, pp.429-444 (Grune and Stratton, New York 1973).

Conway, J. and Lauwers, P.: Hemodynamic and hypotensive effects of long-term therapy with chlorothiazide. Circulation 21: 21-27 (1960).

Conway, J. and Palmero, H.: The vascular effect of the thiazide diuretics. Archives of Internal Medicine 111: 121-207 (1963).

Cooperman, L.B. and Rubin, I.L.: Toxicity of ethacrynic acid and furosemide. American Heart Journal 85: 831-834 (1973).

Costa, G.; Hinsvark, O.N. and Truant, A.P.: Absorption, blood distribution, excretion, and diuretic effect of metolazone. Unpublished observations.

Cutler, R.E.; Forrey, A.W.; Christopher, G. and Kimpel, B.M.: Pharmacokinetics of furosemide in normal subjects and functionally anephric patients. Clinical Pharmacology and Therapeutics 15: 588-596 (1974).

Dargie, H.J.; Collery, C.T. and Daniel, J.: Labetalol in resistant hypertension. British Journal of Clinical Pharmacology 3 (Suppl. 3): 751-755 (1976).

Davies, D.L. and Wilson, G.M.: Diuretics: Mechanism of action and clinical application. Drugs 9: 178-226 (1975).

Day, M.D. and Rand, M.J.: Some observations on the pharmacology of α-methyldopa. British Journal of Pharmacology 22: 72-86 (1964).

Day, M.D.; Roach, A.G. and Whiting, R.L.: The mechanism of the antihypertensive action of α-methyldopa in hypertensive rats. European Journal of Pharmacology 21: 271-280 (1973).

Dollery, C.T.; Davies, D.S.; Draffan, G.H.; Dargie, H.J.; Dean, C.R.; Reid, J.L.; Clare, R.A. and Murray, S.: Clinical pharmacology and pharmacokinetics of clonidine. Clinical Pharmacology and Therapeutics 19: 11-17 (1975).

Dollery, C.T.; Harington, M. and Hodge, J.V.: Haemodynamic studies with methyldopa: Effect on cardiac output and response to pressor amines. British Heart Journal 25: 670-676 (1963).

Domino, E.F.: Drugs affecting behavior; in Di Palma (Ed) Drill's Pharmacology in Medicine, pp.480-488 (Blakiston, New York 1971).

Donald, D.E.; Ferguson, D.A. and Milburn, S.E.: Effect of beta-adrenergic receptor blockade on racing performance of greyhounds with normal and with denervated hearts. Circulation Research 22: 127-134 (1965).

Doyle, A.E.: Use of beta-adrenergic blocking drugs in hypertension. Drugs 8: 422-431 (1974).

Duarte, C.; Winnacker, J.L.; Becker, K.L. and Pace, A.: Thiazide-induced hypercalcemia. New England Journal of Medicine 284: 828-830 (1971).

DuCharme, D.W.; Freyburger, W.A.; Graham, B.E. and Carlson, R.G.: Pharmacologic properties of minoxidil: A new hypotensive agent. J. Pharmacol. Exp. Ther. 184: 662-670 (1973).

Duggan, D.E.: The accumulation of chlorothiazide and related saluretic agents by isolated renal tubules. The Journal of Pharmacology and Experimental Therapeutics 152: 122-129 (1966).

Dustan, H.P.; Cumming, G.R.; Corcoran, A.C. and Page, I.H.: A mechanism of chlorothiazide-enhanced effectiveness of antihypertensive ganglioplegic drugs. Circulation 19: 360-365 (1959).

Dustan, H.P.; Tarazi, R.C. and Bravo, E.L.: Dependence of arterial pressure on intravascular volume in treated hypertensive patients. New England Journal of Medicine 286: 861-866 (1972).

Dustan, H.P.; Tarazi, R.C. and Bravo, E.L.: Diuretic and diet treatment of hypertension. Archives of Internal Medicine 133: 1007-1013 (1974).

Edwards, R.C. and Raftery, E.B.: Haemodynamic effects of long-term oral labetalol. British Journal of Clinical Pharmacology 3 (Suppl. 3): 733-736 (1976).

Editorial: Prazosin and sudden collapse. Lancet 1: 645 (1975a).

Editorial: Rauwolfia and breast cancer. Lancet 2: 312 (1975b).

Editorial: Side effects of practolol. Lancet 1: 289 (1975c).

Elkington, S.G.; Schreiber, W.M. and Conn, H.O.: Hepatic injury caused by L-alpha-emthyldopa. Circulation 40: 589-595 (1969).

Evans, D.A.P. and White, T.A.: Human acetylation polymorphism. Journal of Laboratory and Clinical Medicine 63: 394-403 (1964).

Fann, W.E.; Cavanaugh, J.H.; Kaufmann, J.S.; Griffith, J.D.; Davis, J.M.; Janowsky, D.S. and Oates, J.A.: Doxepin: Effects on transport of biogenic amines in man. Psychopharmacologia 22: 111 (1971).

Feisal, K.A.; Eckstein, J.W.; Horsley, A.W. and Keasling, H.H.: Effects of chlorothiazide on forearm vascular response to norepinephrine. Journal of Applied Physiology 16: 549-552 (1961).

Ferguson, R.K.; Rothenberg, R.J. and Nies, A.S.: Patient acceptance of guanethidine therapy for mild to moderate hypertension: A comparison with reserpine. Circulation 54: 32-37 (1976).

Finch, L. and Haeusler, G.: Further evidence for a central hypotensive action of α-methyldopa in both the rat and cat. British Journal of Pharmacology 47: 217-228 (1973).

Finnerty, F.A., Jr.: Relationship of extracellular fluid volume to the development of drug resistance in the hypertensive patient. American Heart Journal 81: 563-565 (1971).

Fleming, W.L. and Trendelenburg, U.: The development of supersensitivity to norepinephrine after pretreatment with reserpine. Journal of Pharmacology 133: 41-51 (1961).

Ford, R.V.: Clinical pharmacologic investigation of polythiazide, a potent oral diuretic agent. Current Therapeutic Research 3: 320-328 (1961).

Ford, R.V. and Bush, J.: Comparative clinical effects of hydrochlorothiazide and methyclothiazide. Current Therapeutic Research 2: 430-435 (1960).

Franciosa, J.A. and Freis, E.D.: Normal cardiac output during beta-blockade with timolol in hypertensive patients. Clinical Pharmacology and Therapeutics 18: 158-164 (1975).

Franciosa, J.A.; Freis, E.D. and Conway, J.: Antihypertensive and hemodynamic properties of the new beta-adrenergic blocking agent timolol. Circulation 48: 118-124 (1973).

Freis, E.D.: Guanethidine. Progress in Cardiovascular Diseases 8: 183-193 (1965).

Freis, E.D.: Reserpine in hypertension: Present status. American Family Physician 11: 120-122 (1975).

Freis, E.D.; Rose, J.C.; Higgins, T.F.; Finnerty, F.A., Jr.; Kelley, R.T. and Partenope, E.A.: The hemodynamic effects of hypotensive drugs in man. IV. 1-hydrazinophthalazine. Circulation 8: 199-204 (1953).

Freis, E.D.; Wanko, A.; Schnaper, H.W. and Frohlich, E.D.: Mechanism of the altered blood pressure responsiveness produced by chlorothiazide. Journal of Clinical Investigation 39: 1277-1281 (1960).

Frohlich, E.D.; Schnaper, H.W.; Wilson, I.M. and Freis, E.D.: Hemodynamic alterations in hypertensive patients due to chlorothiazide. New England Journal of Medicine 262: 1261-1263 (1960).

Frohlich, E.D.; Tarazi, R.C. and Dustan, H.P.: Peripheral arterial insufficiency. Journal of the American Medical Association 208: 2471-2472 (1969).

Frohlich, E.D.; Tarazi, R.C.; Dustan, H.P. and Page, I.H.: The paradox of beta-adrenergic blockade in hypertension. Circulation 37: 417-423 (1968).

Frohlich, E.D.; Thurman, A.E.; Pfeffer, M.A.; Brobmann, G.F. and Jacobson, E.D.: Altered vascular responsiveness: Initial hypotensive mechanism of thiazide diuretics. Proceedings of the Society for Experimental Biology and Medicine 140: 1190-1196 (1972).

Fuchs, M.; Mallin, S.R.; Irie, S.; Hernando, L. and Moyer, J.H.: A review of the pharmacology and clinical observations of hydrochlorothiazide. Archives of Internal Medicine 105: 30-50 (1960).

Gaffney, T.E.; Chidsey, C.A. and Braunwald, E.: Study of the relationship between the neurotransmitter store and adrenergic nerve block induced by reserpine and guanethidine. Circulation Research 12: 264-268 (1963).

Gavras, H.; Brunner, H.R.; Laragh, J.H.; Sealey, J.E.; Gavras, I. and Vukovich, R.A.: An angiotensin converting-enzyme inhibitor to identify and treat vasoconstrictor and volume factors in hypertensive patients. New England Journal of Medicine 291: 817-821 (1974).

Gavras, H.; Brunner, H.R.; Turini, G.A.; Kershaw, G.R.; Tifft, C.P., Cuttelod, S.; Gavras, I.; Vukovich, R.A. and McKinstry, D.N.: Antihypertensive effect of oral angiotensin converting enzyme inhibitor SQ14225 in man. New England Journal of Medicine 298: 991-995 (1978).

Gifford, R.W., Jr.: Reserpine and guanethidine in the treatment of hypertension; in Onesti, Kim and Moyer (Eds) Hypertension: Mechanisms and Management, pp.305-309 (Grune and Stratton, New York 1973).

Gifford, R.W., Jr.: Clinical application of new antihypertensive drugs. Cleveland Clinic Quarterly 42: 255-262 (1975).

Gifford, R.W., Jr.: Management and treatment of malignant hypertension and hypertensive emergencies; in Genest, Koiw and Kuchel (Eds) Hypertension — Physiopathology and Treatment, pp.1024-1038 (McGraw-Hill, New York 1977).

Gifford, R.W., Jr. and Tarazi, R.C.: Resistant hypertension: Diagnosis and management. Annals of Internal Medicine 88: 661-665 (1978).

Gilder, D.A.; Fain, W. and Simpson, L.L.: A comparison of the abilities of chloropromazine and molindone to interact adversely with guanethidine. Journal of Pharmacology and Experimental Therapeutics 198: 255-263 (1976).

Glontz, G.E. and Saslaw, S.: Methyldopa fever. Archives of Internal Medicine 122: 445-447 (1968).

Goble, A.J.: Diuretics, beta-blockers and vasodilators dosage in mild and moderate hypertension. Medical Journal of Australia (Special Suppl. 1): 14-17 (1975).

Goldberg, A.D.; Wilkinson, P.R. and Raftery, E.B.: The over-shoot phenomenon on withdrawal of clonidine therapy. Postgraduate Medical Journal 52 (Suppl.7): 128-134 (1976).

Goldberg, L.I.; Rick, J.H. and Oparil, S.: Pharmacology of antihypertensive agents, in Genest, Koiw and Kuchel (Eds) Hypertension — Physiopathology and Treatment, pp.1007-1012 (McGraw-Hill, New York 1977).

Goldberg, M.: The renal physiology of diuretics, in Geiger, S.R.: Handbook of Physiology, pp.1003-1031 (American Physiological Society, Washington, DC 1973).

Goldner, M.G.; Zarowitz, H. and Akgun, S.: Hyperglycemia and glycosuria due to thiazide derivatives administered in diabetes mellitus. New England Journal of Medicine 262: 403-405 (1960).

Gottlieb, T.B.; Katz, F.H. and Chidsey, C.A.: Combined therapy with vasodilator drugs and beta-adrenergic blockade in hypertension. A comparative study of minoxidil and hydralazine. Circulation 45: 571-582 (1972).

Gottlieb, T.B.; Thomas, R.C. and Chidsey, C.A.: Pharmacokinetic studies of minoxidil. Clinical Pharmacology and Therapeutics 13: 436-441 (1971).

Graham, R.M.; Muir, M.R. and Hayes, J.M.: Differing effects of the vasodilator drugs, prazosin and diazoxide on plasma renin activity in the dog. Clinical and Experimental Pharmacology and Physiology 3: 1-5 (1976).

Graham, R.M.; Oates, H.F.; Stoker, L.M. and Stokes, G.S.: Alpha blocking action of the antihypertensive agent, prazosin. The Journal of Pharmacology and Experimental Therapeutics 201: 747-752 (1977).

Grayson, M.F.; Smith, A.J. and Smith, R.N.: Absorption, distribution and elimination of ^{14}C-amiloride in normal human subjects. British Journal of Pharmacology 43: 473-474 (1971).

Greither, A.; Goldman, S.; Edelen, J.S.; Cohn, K. and Benet, L.Z.: Erratic and incomplete absorption of furosemide in congestive heart failure (abstract). The American Journal of Cardiology 37: 139 (1976).

Gulati, O.D.; Dave, B.T.; Gokhale, S.D. and Shah, K.M.: Antagonism of adrenergic neuron blockade in hypertensive subjects. Clinical Pharmacology and Therapeutics 7: 510-514 (1965).

Haefely, W.; Hurlimann, A. and Thoenen, H.: The effect of stimulation of sympathetic nerves in the cat treated with reserpine, α-methyldopa and α-methylmetatyrosine. British Journal of Pharmacology 26: 172-185 (1966).

Haeusler, G.: Cardiovascular regulation by central adrenergic mechanisms and its alteration by hypotensive drugs. Circulation Research 36 & 37 (Suppl. 1): 223-232 (1975).

Haggendal, J. and Dahlstrom, A.: The recovery of the capacity for uptake-retention of [^{3}H] noradrenaline in rat adrenergic nerves after reserpine. Journal of Pharmacy and Pharmacology 24: 565-574 (1972).

Hamby, W.M.; Jankowski, G.J.; Pouget, J.M.; Dunea, G. and Gantt, C.L.: Intravenous use of diazoxide in the treatment of severe hypertension. Circulation 37: 169-174 (1968).

Hansson, L.; Hunyor, S.N.; Julius, S. and Hoobler, S.W.: Blood pressure crisis following withdrawal of clonidine with special reference to arterial and urinary catecholamine levels and suggestions for acute management. American Heart Journal 85: 605-610 (1973).

Hansson, L.; Olander, R.; Aberg, H.; Malmcrona, R. and Westerlund, A.: Treatment of hypertension with propranolol and hydralazine. Acta Medica Scandinavica 190: 531-534 (1971).

Hansson, L. and Werko, L.: Beta-adrenergic blockade in hypertension. American Heart Journal 93: 394-402 (1977).

Harber, L.C.; Lashinsky, A.M. and Baer, R.L.: Photosensitivity due to chlorothiazide and hydrochlorothiazide. New England Journal of Medicine 261: 1378-1381 (1959).

Harris, A.L.: Aspects of clonidine therapy. New England Journal of Medicine 294: 845 (1976).

Harrison, D.C.; Chidsey, C.A.; Goldman, R. and Braunwald, E.: Relationships between the release and tissue depletion of norepinephrine from the heart by guanethidine and reserpine. Circulation Research 12: 256-263 (1963).

Hart, L.G. and Schanker, L.S.: Active transport of chlorothiazide into bile. American Journal of Physiology 211: 643-646 (1966).

Hayes, J.M.; Graham, R.M.; O'Connell, B.P.; Muir, M.R.; Speers, E. and Humphery, T.J.: Experience with prazosin in the treatment of patients with severe hypertension. Medical Journal of Australia 1: 562-564 (1976).

Heinonen, O.P.; Shapiro, S.; Tuominen, L. and Turunen, M.I.: Reserpine use in relation to breast cancer. Lancet 2: 675-677 (1974).

Heise, A. and Kronenberg, G.: Alpha-sympathetic receptor stimulation in the brain and hypotensive activity of alpha-methyldopa. European Journal of Pharmacology 17: 315-317 (1972).

Heistad, D.D.; Abboud, F.M. and Ballard, D.R.: Relationship between plasma sodium concentration and vascular reactivity in man. Journal of Clinical Investigation 50: 2022-2032 (1971).

Henning, M.: Studies on the mode of action of α-methyldopa. Acta Physiologica Scandinavica, Suppl. 322 (1969).

Henning, M.: Central action of alpha-methyldopa; in Davies and Reid (Eds) Central Action of Drugs in Blood Pressure Regulation, pp.157-165 (University Park Press, Baltimore 1975).

Hertting, G.; Axelrod, J. and Patrick, R.W.: Actions of bretylium and guanethidine on the uptake and release of [³H] — noradrenaline. British Journal of Pharmacology 18: 161-166 (1962).

Hess, H.J.: Biochemistry and structure-activity studies with prazosin; in Cotton (Ed) Proceedings of a Symposium held at the Centre Interprofessionnel, Geneva, 8 March 1974, pp.3-15 (Elsevier, New York 1974).

Hinsvark, O.N. and Cohen, A.I.: The study of metolazone, a new diuretic, in human body fluids using thin layer separation, liquid chromatographic measurements and ¹⁴C-counting techniques. Federation Proceedings 29: 276 (1970).

Homeida, M.; Jackson, L. and Roberts, C.J.C.: Decreased first-pass metabolism of labetalol in chronic liver disease. British Medical Journal 2: 1048 (1978).

Huang, C.M.; Atkinson, A.J.; Levin, M.; Levin, N.W. and Quintanilla, A.: Pharmacokinetics of furosemide in advanced renal failure. Clinical Pharmacology and Therapeutics 16: 659-666 (1974).

Hutcheon, D.E. and Leonard, G.B.: Therapeutic efficacy of diuretics with different durations of action. Journal of the American Medical Association 185: 640-642 (1963).

Ibsen, H. and Sederberg-Olsen, P.: Changes in glomerular filtration rate during long-term treatment with propranolol in patients with arterial hypertension. Clinical Science 44: 129-134 (1973).

Iggo, A. and Vogt, M.: Preganglionic sympathetic activity in normal and in reserpine-treated cats. Journal of Physiology 150: 114-133 (1960).

Imhof, P.: Characterization of beta-blockers as antihypertensive agents in the light of human pharmacology studies; in Schweizer and Huber (Eds) Beta-blockers: Present Status and Future Prospects, pp.40-50 (University Park Press, Baltimore 1975).

Janis, R.A. and Triggle, D.J.: Effect of diazoxide on aortic reactivity to calcium in spontaneously hypertensive rats. Canadian Journal of Physiology and Pharmacology 51: 621-626 (1973).

Jick, H.; Slone, D.; Shapiro, S. and Heinonen, O.P.: Reserpine and breast cancer. Lancet 2: 669-671 (1974).

Johnson, B.F.: Diazoxide and renal function in man. Clinical Pharmacology and Therapeutics 12: 815-824 (1971).

Johnsson, G. and Regardh, C.G.: Clinical pharmacokinetics of beta-adrenergic blocking drugs. Clinical Pharmacokinetics 1: 233-263 (1976).

Judson, W.E.; Hollander, W. and Wilkins, R.W.: The effects of intravenous Apresoline (hydralazine) on cardiovascular and renal function in patients with and without congestive heart failure. Circulation 13: 664-674 (1956).

Kale, A.K. and Satoskar, R.S.: Modification of the central hypotensive effect of α-methyldopa by reserpine, imipramine and tranylcypromine. European Journal of Pharmacology 9: 120-123 (1970).

Kanada, S.A.; Kanada, D.J.; Hutchinson, R.A. and Wu, D.: Angina-like syndrome with diazoxide therapy for hypertensive crisis. Annals of Internal Medicine 84: 696-699 (1976).

Kane, J.; Gregg, I. and Richards, D.A.: A double-blind trial of labetalol. British Journal of Clinical Pharmacology 3 (Suppl. 3): 737-741 (1976).

Karim, A.; Zagarella, J.; Hribar, J. and Dooley, M.: Spironolactone. I. Disposition and metabolism. Clinical Pharmacology and Therapeutics 19: 158-169 (1976a).

Karim, A.; Zagarella, J.; Hutsell, T.C.; Chao, A. and Baltes, B.J.; Spironolactone, II. Bioavailability. Clinical Pharmacology and Therapeutics 19: 170-176 (1976b).

Karim, A.; Zagarella, J.; Hutsell, T.C. and Dooley, M.: Spironolactone. III. Canrenone-maximum and minimum steady-state plasma levels. Clinical Pharmacology and Therapeutics 19: 177-182 (1976).

Kelly, M.R.; Cutler, R.E., Arden, W.F. and Kimpel, B.M.: Pharmacokinetics of orally administered furosemide. Clinical Pharmacology and Therapeutics 15: 178-186 (1974).

Kennedy, A.C.; Watson, W.C. and Cunningham, C.: The diuretic activity of hydroflumethazide. Lancet 2: 309-131 (1959).

Khatri, I.M. and Cohn, J.N.: Mechanism of exercise hypotension after sympathetic blockade. American Journal of Cardiology 25: 329-338 (1970).

Kim, K.E.; Onesti, G.; Moyer, J.H. and Swartz, C.; Ethacrynic acid and furosemide. The American Journal of Cardiology 27: 407-415 (1971).

Kisin, I. and Yuzhakov, S.: Effects of reserpine, guanethidine and methyldopa on cardiac output and its distribution. European Journal of Pharmacology 35: 253-260 (1976).

Kobinger, W.: Central cardiovascular actions of clonidine; in Davies and Reid (Eds.) Central Action of Drugs in Blood Pressure Regulation, pp.181-193 (University Park Press, Baltimore 1975).

Kobinger, W.: Central modulation of cardiovascular activity by clonidine and other adrenergic substances; in Onesti, Fernandes and Kim (Eds.) Regulation of Blood Pressure by the Central Nervous System, pp.283-292 (Grune and Stratton, New York 1976).

Koch, G.: Haemodynamic effects of combined α- and β-adrenoreceptor blockade after intravenous labetalol in hypertensive patients at rest and during exercise. British Journal of Clinical Pharmacology 3 (Suppl. 3): 725-728 (1976).

Koch-Weser, J.: Myocardial inactivity of therapeutic concentrations of hydralazine and diazoxide. Experientia 30: 170-171 (1974).

Koch-Weser, J.: Hydralazine. New England Journal of Medicine 295: 320-323 (1976a).

Koch-Weser, J.: Diazoxide. New England Journal of Medicine 294: 1271-1274 (1976b).

Kopin, I.J.; Fischer, J.E.; Musacchio, J.M.; Horst, W.D. and Weise, V.K.: "False neurochemical transmitters" and the mechanism of sympathetic blockade by monoamine oxidase inhibitors. Journal of Pharmacology and Experimental Therapeutics 147: 186-193 (1965).

Koshy, M.C.; Mickley, D.; Bourgoignie, J. and Blaufox, M.D.: Physiologic evaluation of a new antihypertensive agent. Prazosin HCl. Circulation 55: 533-537 (1977).

Kosman, M.E.: Evaluation of clonidine hydrochloride (Catapres). A new antihypertensive agent. Journal of the American Medical Association 233: 174-176 (1975).

Kwan, K.C.; Foltz, E.L.; Breault, G.O.; Baer, J.E. and Totaro, J.A.: Pharmacokinetics of methyldopa in man. Journal of Pharmacology and Experimental Therapeutics 198: 264-277 (1976).

Landesman, R.; Coutinho, E.M.; Wilson, K.H. et al.: The relaxant effect of diazoxide on non gravid human myometrium in vivo. American Journal of Obstetrics and Gynecology 102: 1080-1084 (1968).

Lant, A.F. and Wilson, G.M.: Diuretics, in Black (Ed): Renal Disease, p.655 (Blackwell, Oxford 1972).

Laska, E.M.; Siegel, C.; Meisner, M.; Fischer, S. and Wanderling, J.: Matched-pairs study of reserpine use and breast cancer. Lancet 2: 296-300 (1975).

Lassen, J.B. and Nielsen, O.E.: Investigations into the diuretic effect and elimination of triamterene. Acta Pharmacologica et Toxicologica 20: 309-316 (1963).

Lee, W.C. and Shideman, F.E.: Inotropic action of hexamethonium. Circulation Research 6: 66-71 (1958).

Leonard, J.W.; Gifford, R.W., Jr. and Humphrey, D.C.: Treatment of hypertension with methyldopa alone or combined with diuretics and/or guanethidine. American Heart Journal 69: 610-618 (1965).

Lertora, J.J.L.; Mark, A.L.; Johannsen, U.J.; Wilson, W.R. and Abboud, F.M.: Selective beta-1 receptor blockade with oral practolol in man. A dose-related phenomenon. Journal of Clinical Investigation 56: 719-724 (1975).

Lesser, J.M.; Israili, Z.H.; Davis, E. and Dayton, P.G.: Fate of hydralazine-^{14}C in man and dog. Clinical Pharmacology and Therapeutics 14: 140 (1973).

Lesser, J.M.; Israili, Z.H.; Davis, D.C. and Dayton, P.G.: Metabolism and disposition of hydralazine-^{14}C in man and dog. Drug Metabolism and Disposition 2: 351-360 (1974).

Leth, A.: Changes in plasma and extracellular fluid volumes in patients with essential hypertension during long-term treatment with hydrochlorothiazide. Circulation 42: 479-485 (1970).

Levine, R.J. and Sjoerdsma, A.: Dissociation of the decarboxylase-inhibiting and norepinephrine-depleting effects of α-methyldopa, 4-bromo-3-hydroxybenzyloxyamine and related substances. Journal of Pharmacology and Experimental Therapeutics 146: 42-47 (1964).

Lewis, P.J.: Propranolol — an antihypertensive drug with a central action; in Davies and Reid (Eds) Central Action of Drugs in Blood Pressure Regulation, pp.206-224 (University Park Press, Baltimore 1975).

Lockwood, C.H.; Nicholls, D.M.; Tropp, V.L. and Lewis, J.A.: Diazoxide therapy in hypertension. American Journal of the Medical Sciences 246: 312-318 (1963).

Lowder, S.C. and Liddle, G.W.: Effects of guanethidine and methyldopa on a standardized test for renin responsiveness. Annals of Internal Medicine 82: 757-760 (1975).

Lund-Johansen, P.: Hemodynamic changes in long-term diuretic therapy of essential hypertension. Acta Medica Scandinavica 187: 509-518 (1970).

Lund-Johansen, P.: Hemodynamic changes at rest and during exercise in long-term prazosin therapy for essential hypertension. Clinical Symposium Proceedings, Postgraduate Medicine, pp.45-52 (November, 1975).

Lund-Johansen, P.: Hemodynamic effects of clonidine in man; in Onesti, Fernandes and Kim (Eds) Regulation of Blood Pressure by the Central Nervous System, pp.355-365 (Grune and Stratton, New York 1976).

Lydtin, H.; Kusus, T.; Daniel, W.; Schierl, W.; Ackenheil, M.; Kempter, H.; Lohmoller, G.; Miklas, M. and Walter, I.: Propranolol therapy in essential hypertension. American Heart Journal 83: 589-595 (1972).

Lyons, H.; Pinn, V.W.; Cortell, S.; Cohen, J.J. and Harrington, J.T.: Allergic interstitial nephritis causing reversible renal failure in four patients with idiopathic nephrotic syndrome. New England Journal of Medicine 288: 124-128 (1973).

MacCarthy, E.P.; Frost, G.W. and Stokes, G.S.: Labetalol in hypertensive emergencies. Medical Journal of Australia 1: 399 (1978).

McMartin, C.; Rondel, R.K.; Vinter, J.; Allan, B.R.; Humberstone, M.; Leishman, A.W.D.; Sandler, G.

and Thirkettle, J.L.: The fate of guanethidine in two hypertensive patients. Clinical Pharmacology and Therapeutics 11: 423-431 (1970).

McMartin, C. and Simpson, P.: The absorption and metabolism of guanethidine in hypertensive patients requiring different doses of the drug. Clinical Pharmacology and Therapeutics 12: 73-77 (1971).

Mack, T.M.; Henderson, B.E.; Gerkins, V.R.; Arthur, M.; Baptista, J. and Pike, M.C.: Reserpine and breast cancer in a retirement community. New England Journal of Medicine 292: 1366-1370 (1975).

Marquez-Julio, A. and Uldall, P.R.: Pericardial effusions associated with minoxidil. Lancet 2: 816 (1977).

Marshall, A.J.; Barritt, D.W.; Pocock, J. and Heaton, S.T.: Evaluation of β-blockade, bendrofluazide and prazosin in severe hypertension. Lancet 1: 271 (1977).

Mathog, R.H. and Klein, W.J.: Ototoxicity of ethacrynic acid and aminoglycoside antibiotics in uremia. New England Journal of Medicine 280: 1223-1224 (1969).

Mathog, R.H.; Thomas, W.G. and Hudson, W.R.: Ototoxicity of new and potent diuretics. Archives of Otolaryngology 92: 7-13 (1970).

Mees, E.J.D. and Geyskes, G.G.: A comparative study of the diuretics chlorthalidonum and cyclopenthiazidum. Acta Medica Scandinavica 175: 703-713 (1964).

Mendlowitz, M.; Naftchi, N.; Gitlow, S.E.; Weinreb, L. and Wolf, R.L.: The effect of chlorothiazide and its congeners on the digital circulation in normotensive subjects and in patients with essential hypertension. Annals of the New York Academy of Sciences 88: 964-974 (1960).

Meyer, J.S.; Savada, R.; Kitamura, A. and Toyoda, M.: Cerebral blood flow after control of hypertension in stroke. Neurology 18: 772 (1968).

Michelakis, A.N. and McAllister, R.G.: The effect of chronic adrenergic receptor blockade on plasma renin activity in man. Journal of Clinical Endocrinology and Metabolism 34: 386-394 (1972).

Miller, A.C. and Reid, W.M.: Methyldopa-induced granulomatous hepatitis. Journal of the American Medical Association 235: 2001-2002 (1976).

Miller, R.R.; Awan, N.A.; Maxwell, K.S. and Mason, D.T.: Sustained reduction of cardiac impedance and preload in congestive heart failure with the antihypertensive vasodilator prazosin. New England Journal of Medicine 297: 303-307 (1977).

Miller, R.R.; Vismara, L.A.; Zelis, R.; Amsterdam, E.A. and Mason, D.T.: Clinical use of sodium nitroprusside in chronic ischemic heart disease. Effects on peripheral vascular resistance and venous tone and on ventricular volume, pump and mechanical performance. Circulation 51: 328-336 (1975).

Miller, W.E.; Gifford, R.W., Jr.; Humphrey, D.C. and Vidt, D.G.: Management of severe hypertension with intravenous injections of diazoxide. American Journal of Cardiology 24: 870-875 (1969).

Mitchell, J.R. and Oates, J.A.: Guanethidine and related agents. I. Mechanism of the selective blockade of adrenergic neurons and its antagonism by drugs. Journal of Pharmacology and Experimental Therapeutics 172: 100-197 (1970).

Mitchell, J.R.; Cavanaugh, J.H.; Arias, L. and Oates, J.A.: Guanethidine and related agents. III. Antagonism by drugs which inhibit the norepinephrine pump in man. Journal of Clinical Investigation 49: 1596-1604 (1970).

Mohammed, S.; Gaffney, T.E.; Yard, A.C. and Gomez, H.: Effect of methyldopa, reserpine and guanethidine on hindleg vascular resistance. Journal of Pharmacology and Experimental Therapeutics 160: 300-307 (1968).

Mohammed, S.; Fasola, A.; Privitera, P.J.; Lipicky, R.J.; Martz, B.L. and Gaffney, T.E.: Effect of methyldopa on plasma renin activity in man. Circulation Research 25: 543-548 (1969).

Mookerjee, S.; Eich, R.H.; Obeid, A.I. and Smulyan, H.: Hemodynamic and plasma renin effects of propranolol in essential hypertension. Archives of Internal Medicine 137: 290-295 (1977).

Moore-Jones, S. and Perry, H.M.: Radioautographic localization of hydralazine-1-C^{14} in arterial walls. Proceedings of the Society for Experimental Biology and Medicine 122: 576-579 (1966).

Morgan, T.O.; Robert, R.; Carney, S.L.; Louis, W.J. and Doyle, A.E.: Beta-adrenergic receptor blocking drugs, hypertension and plasma renin. Journal of Clinical Pharmacology 2: 159-164 (1975).

Morgan, T.O.; Sabto, J.; Anavekar, S.N.; Louis, W.J. and Doyle, A.E.: A comparison of beta-adrenergic blocking drugs in the treatment of hypertension. Postgraduate Medical Journal 50: 253-259 (1974).

Moyer, J.H. and Brest, A.N.: Hydralazine in the treatment of hypertension. Medical Clinics of North America 45: 375-383 (1961).

Mroczek, W.J.; Leibel, B.A.; Davidov, M. and Finnerty, F.A., Jr.: The importance of the rapid administration of diazoxide in accelerated hypertension. New England Journal of Medicine 285: 603-606 (1971).

Mudge, G.H.: Diuretics and other agents employed in the mobilization of edema fluid, in Goodman and Gilman (Eds) The Pharmacological Basis of Therapeutics, pp.817-847 (MacMillian, New York 1975).

Murphy, J.; Casey, W. and Lasagna, L.: The effect of dosage regimen on the diuretic efficacy of chlorothiazide in human subjects. Journal of Pharmacology and Experimental Therapeutics 134: 286-290 (1961).

Muscholl, E. and Maitre, L.: Release by sympathetic stimulation of α-methylcoradrenaline stored in the heart after administration of α-methyldopa. Experientia 19: 658-659 (1964).

Myers, M.G. and Hope-Gill, H.F.: Effect of d-propranolol on glucose-stimulated insulin release. Clinical Research 25: 683A (1977).

Myers, M.G.; Lewis, P.J.; Reid, J.L. and Dollery, C.T.: Brain concentration of propranolol in relation to hypotensive effect in the rabbit with observations on brain propranolol levels in man. Journal of Pharmacology and Experimental Therapeutics 192: 327-335 (1975).

Myhre, E.; Stenbaek, O.; Brodwall, E.K. and Hansen, T.: Conjugation of methyldopa in renal failure. Scandinavian Journal of Clinical and Laboratory Investigation 29: 195-204 (1972b).

Myhre, E.; Brodwall, E.K.: Stenbaek, O. and Hansen, T.: Plasma turnover of methyldopa in advanced renal failure. Acta Medica Scandinavica 191: 343-347 (1972a).

Niarchos, A.P. and Tarazi, R.C.: Hemodynamic effects of beta-adrenergic blocking agents in hypertension; in Onesti, Fernandes and Kim (Eds) Regulation of Blood Pressure by the Central Nervous System, pp.397-409 (Grune and Stratton, New York 1976).

Nickerson, M. and Collier, B.: Drugs inhibiting adrenergic nerves and structures innervated by them; in Goodman and Gilman (Eds) The Pharmacological Basis of Therapeutics, 5th ed., pp.557-559 (MacMillan, New York 1975).

Nickerson, M. and Ruedy, M.: Antihypertensive agents and the drug therapy of hypertension; in Goodman and Gilman (Eds) The Pharmacological Basis of Therapeutics, 5th ed., pp.705-726 (MacMillan, New York 1975).

Nies, A.S. and Shand, D.G.: Hypertensive response to propranolol in a patient treated with methyldopa — a proposed mechanism. Clinical Pharmacology and Therapeutics 14: 823-826 (1973).

Nies, A.S. and Shand, D.G.: Clinical pharmacology of propranolol. Circulation 52: 6-51 (1975).

Oates, J.A.; Gillespie, L.; Udenfriend, S. and Sjoerdsma, A.: Decarboxylase inhibition and blood pressure reduction by α-methyl-3,4-dihydroxy-DL-phenylalanine. Science 31: 1890-1891 (1960).

Oates, J.A.; Mitchell, J.R.; Feagin, O.T.; Kaufmann, J.S. and Shand, D.G.: Distribution of guanidinium antihypertensives — mechanism of their selective action. Annals of the New York Academy of Sciences 179: 302-309 (1971).

O'Fallon, W.M.; Labarthe, D.R. and Kurland, L.T.: Rauwolfia derivatives and breast cancer. Lancet 2: 292-300 (1975).

Ogilvie, R.I. and Schlieper, E.: The effect of hydrochlorothiazide on venous reactivity in hypertensive man. Clinical Pharmacology and Therapeutics 11: 589-594 (1970).

O'Malley, K.; Segal, J.L.; Israili, Z.H.; Boles, M.; McNay, J.L. and Dayton, P.G.: Duration of hydralazine action in hypertension. Clinical Pharmacology and Therapeutics 18: 581-586 (1975a).

O'Malley, K.; Velasco, M.; Wells, J. and McNay, J.L.: Control plasma renin activity and changes in sympathetic tone as determinants of minoxidil-induced increase in plasma renin activity. Journal of Clinical Investigation 55: 230-235 (1975b).

O'Malley, K.; Velasco, M.; Wells, J. and McNay, J.: Mechanism of the interaction of propranolol and a potent vasodilator antihypertensive agent — minoxidil. European Journal of Clinical Pharmacology 9: 355-360 (1976).

Ondetti, M.A.; Rubin, B. and Cushman, D.W.: Design of specific inhibitors of angiotensin-converting enzyme: New class of orally active antihypertensive agents. Science 196: 441-444 (1977).

Onesti, G.: Systemic hemodynamic effects of α-methyldopa in man; in Onesti, Fernandes and Kim (Eds) Regulation of Blood Pressure by the Central Nervous System, pp.387-396 (Grune and Stratton, New York 1976).

Onesti, G.; Brest, A.N.; Novack, P.; Kasparian, H. and Moyer, J.H.: Pharmacodynamic effects of alpha-methyldopa in hypertensive subjects. American Heart Journal 67: 32-38 (1964).

Onesti, G.; Kim, K.E.; Swartz, C. and Moyer, J.H.: Hemodynamic effects of antihypertensive agents; in Onesti, Kim and Moyer (Eds) Hypertension: Mechanisms and Management, pp.227-240 (Grune and Stratton, New York 1973).

Onesti, G.; Schwartz, A.B.; Kim, K.E.; Paz-Martinez, V. and Swartz, C.: Antihypertensive effect of clonidine. Circulation Research 28 & 29 (Suppl. 2): 53-69 (1971).

Onesti, G.; Schwartz, A.B.; Kim, K.E.; Swartz, C. and Brest, A.N.: Pharmacodynamic effects of a new antihypertensive drug, Catapres (ST-155). Circulation 39: 219-228 (1969).

Page, I.H.; Hurley, R.E. and Dustan, H.P.: The prolonged treatment of hypertension with guanethidine. Journal of the American Medical Association 175: 543-549 (1961).

Palmer, R.J. and Lasseter, K.C.: Sodium nitroprusside. N. Eng. J. Med. 292: 294-297 (1975).

Perry, H.M.: A method of quantitating 1-hydrazinophthalazine in body fluids. Journal of Laboratory and Clinical Medicine 41: 566-595 (1953).

Perry, H.M.: Late toxicity to hydralazine resembling systemic lupus erythematosus or rheumatoid arthritis. American Journal of Medicine 54: 58-72 (1973).

Perry, H.M.; Comens, P. and Yunice, A.: Distribution of hydralazine-1-C^{14} after injection into normal mice. Journal of Laboratory and Clinical Medicine 59: 456-461 (1972).

Perry, H.M.; Tan, E.M.; Carmody, S. and Sakamoto, A.: Relationship of acetyltransferase activity to antinuclear antibodies and toxic symptoms in hypertensive patients treated with hydralazine. Journal of Laboratory and Clinical Medicine 76: 114-125 (1970).

Peters, G. and Roch-Ramel, F.: Thiazide diuretics and related drugs, in Eichler, Farah, Herken and Welch (Eds) Handbook of Experimental Pharmacology Vol. 24, pp. 257-278 (Springer Verlag, New York 1969).

Pettinger, W.A.: Clonidine, a new antihypertensive drug. New England Journal of Medicine 293: 1179-1180 (1975).

Pettinger, W.A. and Mitchel, H.C.: Minoxidil — an alternative to nephrectomy for refractory hypertension. New England Journal of Medicine 289: 167-171 (1973).

Piala, J.J.; Poutsiaka, J.W.; Smith, C.I.; Burke, J.C. and Craver, B.N.: Pharmacology of benzydroflumethiazide (naturetin). Journal of Pharmacology and Experimental Therapeutics 134: 273-280 (1961).

Pinson, R., Jr.; Schreiber, E.C.; Wiseman, E.H.; Chiaini, J. and Baumgartner, D.: The fate and excretion of polythiazide in the dog. Journal of Medicinal and Pharmaceutical Chemistry 5: 491-503 (1962).

Podolsky, S. and Pattavina, C.: Hyperosmolar nonketonic diabetic coma: A complication of propranolol therapy. Metabolism 22: 685-693 (1973).

Prescott, L.F.; Buhs, R.P.; Beattie, J.O.; Speth, O.C.; Trenner, N.R. and Lasagna, L.: Combined clinical and metabolic study of the effects of alphamethyldopa on hypertensive patients. Circulation 34: 308-321 (1966).

Prichard, B.N.C. and Boakes, A.J.: Labetalol in long-term treatment of hypertension. British Journal of Clinical Pharmacology 3 (Suppl. 3): 743-750 (1976).

Prichard, B.N.C., Thompson, F.O.; Boakes, A.J. and Joekes, A.M.: Some haemodynamic effects of compound AH5158 compared with propranolol, propranolol plus hydrallazine and diazoxide: The use of AH5158 in the treatment of hypertension. Clinical Science and Molecular Medicine 48: 975 (1975).

Pruitt, A.W.; Winkel, J.S. and Dayton, P.G.: Variations in the fate of triamterene. Clinical Pharmacology and Therapeutics 21: 610-619 (1977).

Puig, M.; Wakade, A.R. and Kirpekar, S.M.: Effect on the sympathetic nervous system of chronic treatment with pargyline and 1-dopa. The Journal of Pharmacology and Experimental Therapeutics 182: 130-134 (1972).

Pulver, R.; Wirz, H. and Stenger, E.G.: Uber das Verhalten des Diureticums Hygroton (G 33 182) im Stoffwechsel. Schweizerische Medizinische Wochenschrift 43: 1130-1133 (1959).

Putzeys, M.R. and Hoobler, S.W.: Comparison of clonidine and methyldopa on blood pressure and side effects in hypertensive patients. American Heart Journal 83: 464-468 (1972).

Quetsch, R.M.; Achor, R.W.P.; Litin, E.M. and Faucett, R.L.: Depressive reactions in hypertensive patients. A comparison of those treated with Rauwolfia and those receiving no specific antihypertensive treatment. Circulation 19: 366-375 (1959).

Ramsay, L.; Asbury, M.; Shelton, J. and Harrison, I.: Spironolactone and canrenoate-K: relative potency at steady state. Clinical Pharmacology and Therapeutics 21: 602-609 (1977).

Rehbinder, V.D. and Deckers, W.: Utersuchungen zur pharmakokinetik und zum metabolismus des 2-(2,6-Dichlorphenylamino)-2-imidazolin-hydrochlorid (St 155). Arzneimittel-Forschung 19: 169-176 (1969).

Reid, I.A.; MacDonald, D.M.; Pachnis, B. and Ganong, W.F.: Studies concerning the mechanism of suppression of renin secretion by clonidine. Journal of Pharmacology and Experimental Therapeutics 192: 713-721 (1975).

Reidenberg, M.M.; Drayer, D.; DeMarco, A.L. and Bello, C.T.: Hydralazine elimination in man. Clinical Pharmacology and Therapeutics 14: 970-977 (1973).

Reubi, F.C.: Clinical use of furosemide. Annals of the New York Academy of Sciences 139: 433-442 (1966).

Reubi, F.C. and Cottier, P.T.: Effects of reduced glomerular filtration rate on responsiveness to chlorothiazide and mercurial diuretics. Circulation 23: 200-210 (1961).

Reusch, C.S.: The cardiorenal hemodynamic effects of antihypertensive therapy with reserpine. American Heart Journal 64: 643-649 (1962).

Richards, D.A.: Pharmacological effects of labetalol in man. British Journal of Clinical Pharmacology 3 (Suppl. 3): 721-723 (1976).

Richardson, D.W. and Wyso, E.M.: Human pharmacology of guanethidine. Annals of the New York Academy of Sciences 88: 944-955 (1960).

Richardson, D.W.; Wyso, E.M.; Magee, J.H. and Cavell, G.C.: Circulatory effects of guanethidine: Clinical, renal and cardiac responses to treatment with a novel antihypertensive drug. Circulation 22: 184-190 (1960).

Robson, A.O.; Ashcroft, R.; Kerr, D.N.S. and Teasdale, G.: The diuretic response to frusemide. Lancet 2: 1085-1088 (1964).

Rønne-Rasmussen, J.O.; Andersen, G.S.; Bowal Jensen, N. and Andersson, E.: Acute effect of intravenous labetalol in the treatment of systemic arterial hypertension. British Journal of Clinical Pharmacology 3 (Suppl. 3): 805-808 (1976).

Rose, H.J.; O'Malley, K. and Pruitt, A.W.: Depression of renal clearance of furosemide in man by azotemia. Clinical Pharmacology and Therapeutics of 21: 141-146 (1977).

Rosei, E.A.; Brown, J.J.; Lever, A.F. and Robertson, A.S.: Treatment of phaeochromocytoma and of clonidine withdrawal hypertension with labetalol. British Journal of Clinical Pharmacology 3 (Suppl. 3): 809-815 (1976).

Rowe, G.C.; Huston, J.H.; Maxwell, G.M.; Crosley, A.P. and Crumpton, C.W.: Hemodynamic effects of

1-hydrazinophthalazine in patients with arterial hypertension. Journal of Clinical Investigation 34: 115-120 (1965).

Rubin, A.A.; Roth, F.E.; Taylor, R.M. and Rosenkilde, H.: Pharmacology of diazoxide, an antihypertensive, non-diuretic benzothiadiazine. Journal of Pharmacology and Experimental Therapeutics 136: 344-352 (1962).

Rupp, W.: Pharmacokinetics and pharmacodynamics of lasix. Scottish Medical Journal 19 (Suppl 1): 5-13 (1974).

Rutledge, C.O. and Weiner, N.: The effect of reserpine upon the synthesis of norepinephrine in the isolated rabbit heart. Journal of Pharmacology and Experimental Therapeutics 157: 290-302 (1967).

Sadee, W.; Abshagen, U.; Finn, C. and Rietbrock, N.: Conversion of spironolactone to canrenone and disposition kinetics of spironolactone and canrenoate-potassium in rats. Naunyn-Schmidedberg's Archives of Pharmacology 283: 303-318 (1974).

Sadee, W.; Dagcioglu, M. and Schroder, R.: Pharmacokinetics of spironolactone, canrenone and canrenoate-K in humans. The Journal of Pharmacology and Experimental Therapeutics 185: 686-695 (1973).

Sannerstedt, R.: Haemodynamic effects of adrenergic beta-receptor-blocking agents in arterial hypertension; in Berglund, Hansson and Werko (Eds) Pathophysiology and Management of Arterial Hypertension, p.194 (Lingdren and Soner, Stockholm 1975).

Sannerstedt, R. and Conway, J.: Hemodynamic and vascular responses to antihypertensive treatment with adrenergic blocking agents: A review. American Heart Journal 79: 122-127 (1970).

Sannerstedt, R.; Stenberg, J.; Vedin, A.; Wilhelmsson, C. and Werko, L.: Chronic beta-adrenergic blockade in arterial hypertension. American Journal of Cardiology 29: 718-798 (1972).

Sannerstedt, R.; Stenberg, J.; Johnsson, G. and Werko, L.: Hemodynamic interference of alprenolol with dihydralazine in normal and hypertensive man. American Journal of Cardiology 28: 316-320 (1971).

Schwartz, G.H.; David, D.S.; Riggio, R.R.; Stenzel, K.H. and Rubin, A.L.: Ototoxicity induced by furosemide. The New England Journal of Medicine 282: 1413-1414 (1970).

Scriabine, A.; Schreiber, E.C.; Yu, M. and Wiseman, E.H.: Renal clearance of polythiazide. Proceedings of the Society of Experimental Biology and Medicine 110: 872-875 (1962).

Sellars, E.M. and Koch-Weser, J.: Protein binding and vascular activity of diazoxide. New England Journal of Medicine 281: 1141-1144 (1969).

Shah, P.K.: Ventricular unloading in the management of heart disease: Role of vasodilators. Part I. American Heart Journal 93: 256-260 (1977).

Shand, D.G.: Pharmacokinetic properties of the beta-adrenergic receptor blocking drugs. Drugs 7: 39-47 (1974).

Shand, D.G.; Morgan, D.H. and Oates, J.A.: The release of guanethidine and bethanidine by splenic nerve stimulation: A quantitative evaluation showing dissociation from adrenergic blockade. Journal of Pharmacology and Experimental Therapeutics 184: 73-80 (1973).

Shand, D.G.; Nies, A.S.; McAllister, R.G. and Oates, J.A.: A loading-maintenance regimen for more rapid initiation of the effect of guanethidine. Clinical Pharmacology and Therapeutics 18: 139-144 (1975).

Shapiro, A.P.; Benedek, T.G. and Small, J.L.: Effect of thiazides on carbohydrate metabolism in patients with hypertension. New England Journal of Medicine 265: 1028-1033 (1961).

Sheppard, H.; Mowles, T.F.; Bowen, N.; Renzi, A.A. and Plummer, A.J.: Distribution and fate of hydrochlorothiazide-H^3. Toxicology and Applied Pharmacology 2: 188-194 (1960).

Shore, P.A.: Transport and storage of biogenic amines. Annual Review of Pharmacology 12: 209-226 (1972).

Simpson, F.O.: Beta-adrenergic receptor blocking drugs in hypertension. Drugs 7: 85-105 (1974).

Sjoerdsma, A.; Vendsaly, A. and Engelman, K.: Studies on the metabolism and mechanism of action of methyldopa. Circulation 28: 492-502 (1963).

Smith, A.J.: Clinical features of fluid retention complicating treatment with guanethidine. Circulation 31: 485-489 (1965a).

Smith, A.J.: Fluid retention produced by guanethidine. Changes in body exchangeable sodium, blood volume, and creatinine clearance. Circulation 31: 490-496 (1965b).

Sourkes, T.L.: Inhibition of dihydroxyphenylalanine decarboxylase by derivatives of phenylalanine. Archives of Biochemistry and Biophysics 51: 444-456 (1954).

Steinmuller, S.R. and Puschett, J.B.: Effects of metolazone in man: comparison with chlorothiazide. Kidney International 1: 169-181 (1972).

Stone, C.A.; Porter, C.C.; Stavorski, J.M.; Ludden, C.T. and Totaro, J.A.: Antagonism of certain effects of catecholamine depleting agents by antidepressant and related drugs. Journal of Pharmacology and Experimental Therapeutics 144: 196-204 (1964).

Strandberg, I.; Boman, G.; Hassler, L. and Sjoqvist, F.: Acetylator phenotype in patients with hydralazine-induced lupoid syndrome. Acta Medica Scandinavica 200: 367-371 (1976).

Streeten, D.H.P.; Dalakos, T.G.; Anderson, G.H. and Freiberg, J.M.: Use of angiotensin II analogs and converting enzyme inhibitors in management of hypertension; in Genest, Koiw and Kuchel (Eds) Hypertension — Physiopathology and Treatment, pp.1127-1134 (McGraw-Hill, New York 1977).

Streeten, D.H.P.; Dalakos, T.G.; Anderson, G.H. and Freiberg, J.M.: Use of angiotensin II analogs and converting enzyme inhibitors in management of hypertension; in Genest, Koiw and Kuchel (Eds.) Hypertension, pp.1127-1134 (McGraw-Hill, New York 1977).

Stunkard, A.; Wertheimer, L. and Redisch, W.: Studies on hydralazine; evidence for a peripheral site of action. Journal of Clinical Investigation 33: 1047-1053 (1954).

Sundquist, H.; Anttila, M. and Arstila, M.: Antihypertensive effects of practolol and sotalol. Clinical Pharmacology and Therapeutics 16: 465-472 (1974).

Surveyor, I.; Evans, B.; Saunders, K.C. and Parry, T.E.: Autoimmune haemolytic anaemia complicating methyldopa therapy. Postgraduate Medical Journal 44: 438-442 (1968).

Swainson, C.P. and Winney, R.J.: Effect of beta-blockade in chronic renal failure. British Medical Journal 1: 459 (1976).

Swartz, C.; Seller, R.; Fuchs, M.; Brest, A.N. and Moyer, J.H.: Five years' experience with the evaluation of diuretic agents. Circulation 28: 1042-1049 (1963).

Suki, W.; Dawoud, F.; Eknoyan, G. and Martinez-Maldonado, M.: Effects of metolazone on renal function in normal man. The Journal of Pharmacology and Experimental Therapeutics 180: 6-12 (1972).

Suki, W.; Rector, F.C. and Seldin, D.W.: The site of action of furosemide and other sulfonamide diuretics in the dog. Journal of Clinical Investigation 44: 1458-1469 (1965).

Talseth, T.: Studies on hydralazine. I. Serum concentration of hydralazine in man after a single dose and at steady state. European Journal of Clinical Pharmacology 10: 183-187 (1976a).

Talseth, T.: Studies on hydralazine. II. Elimination rate and steady-state concentration in patients with impaired renal function. European Journal of Clinical Pharmacology 10: 311-317 (1976b).

Talseth, T.: Studies on hydralazine. III. Bioavailability of hydralazine in man. European Journal of Clinical Pharmacology 10: 395-401 (1976c).

Tarazi, R.C.: Diuretic drugs: Mechanisms of antihypertensive action; in Onesti, Kim and Moyer (Eds) Hypertension: Mechanisms and Management, pp.251-260 (Grune and Stratton, New York 1973a).

Tarazi, R.C.: Long-term hemodynamic effects of beta-adrenergic blockade in hypertension; in Onesti, Kim and Moyer (Eds.) Hypertension: Mechanisms and Management, pp.343-349 (Grune and Stratton, New York 1973b).

Tarazi, R.C. and Dustan, H.P.: Beta-adrenergic blockade in hypertension. American Journal of Cardiology 29: 633-640 (1972).

Tarazi, R.C. and Dustan, H.P.: Neurogenic participation in essential and renovascular hypertension assessed by acute ganglionic blockade. Correlation with haemodynamic indices and intravascular volume. Clinical Science 44: 197-212 (1973).

Tarazi, R.C. and Dustan, H.P.: Hemodynamic effects of diuretics in hypertension. Contributions to Nephrology 8: 162-170 (1977).

Tarazi, R.C. and Gifford, R.W., Jr.: Drug treatment of hypertension; in Donoso (Ed) Drugs in Cardiology, pp.1-41 (Stratton Intercontinental, New York 1975).

Tarazi, R.C.; Dustan, H.P. and Bravo, E.L.: Haemodynamic effects of propranolol in hypertension: A review. Postgraduate Medical Journal 52: 92-100 (1976).

Tarazi, R.C.; Dustan, H.P.; Bravo, E.L. and Niarchos, A.P.: Vasodilating drugs: Contrasting haemodynamic effects. Clinical Science and Molecular Medicine 51 (Suppl. 3): 575-578 (1977a).

Tarazi, R.C.; Dustan, H.P. and Frohlich, E.D.: Long-term thiazide therapy in essential hypertension. Circulation 41: 709-717 (1970).

Tarazi, R.C.; Ferrario, C.M. and Dustan, H.P.: The heart in hypertension; in Genest, Koiw and Kuchel (Eds) Hypertension — Physiopathology and Treatment, pp.738-754 (McGraw-Hill, New York 1977b).

Taylor, R.M. and Maren, T.H.: The pharmacology of trichlormethiazide, a benzothiadiazine diuretic. Journal of Pharmacology and Experimental Therapeutics 140: 249-257 (1963).

Thirwell, M.P. and Zsoter, T.T.: The effect of diazoxide on the veins. American Heart Journal 83: 512-517 (1972).

Thompson, F.D. and Joekes, A.M.: Beta-blockade in the presence of renal disease and hypertension. British Medical Journal 1: 555-556 (1974).

Thornton, W.E.: Dementia induced by methyldopa with haloperidol. New England Journal of Medicine 295: 1222 (1976).

Trinker, F.R.: The significance of the relative potencies of noradrenaline and α-methylnoradrenaline for the mode of action of α-methyldopa. Journal of Pharmacy and Pharmacology 23: 306-308 (1971).

Turner, A.S.; Watson, O.F. and Brocklehurst, J.E.: Prazosin in hypertension. Clinical studies with special reference to initiation of therapy. Australian Medical Journal 2 (Special Suppl.): 33 (1977).

Turner, A.S.; Watson, O. and Peel, J.S.: Clinical experience with prazosin hydrochloride in arterial hypertension. New Zealand Medical Journal 81: 240-242 (1975).

Tweeddale, M.G. and Ogilvie, R.I.: Antagonism of spironolactone-induced natriuresis by aspirin in man. New England Journal of Medicine 289: 198-200 (1973).

Tweeddale, M.G. and Ogilvie, R.I.: Improved method for estimating chlorthalidone in body fluids. Journal of Pharmaceutical Sciences 63: 1065-1067 (1974).

Ueda, H.; Kaneko, Y.; Takeda, T.; Ikeda, T. and Yagi, S.: Observations on the mechanism of renin release by hydralazine in hypertensive patients. Circulation Reserach 26 & 27 (Suppl. 2): 201-206 (1970).

VanderKolk, K.; Dontas, A.S. and Hoobler, S.W.: Renal and hypotensive effects of acute and chronic oral treatment with 1-hydrazinophthalazine (Apresoline) in hypertension. American Heart Journal 48: 95-101 (1954).

van Zwieten, P.A.: The central action of antihypertensive drugs, mediated via central α-receptors. Journal of Pharmacy and Pharmacology 25: 89-95 (1973).

van Zwieten, P.A.: Interaction between centrally acting hypertensive drugs and tricyclic antidepressants. Archives Internationales de Pharmacodynamie et de Therapie. 214: 12-30 (1975).

van Zwieten, P.A.: Centrally mediated action of α-methyldopa; in Onesti, Fernandes and Kim (Eds) Regulation of Blood Pressure by the Central Nervous System, pp.293-301 (Grune and Stratton, New York 1976).

van Zwieten, P.A.: Interactions interfering with central adrenoreceptor activity and hypotension of centrally acting antihypertensive agents. Progress in Brain Research, 47: 385-390 (1977).

Venables, R.L. and Duff, R.S.: A comparative trial of prazosin and methyldopa. In Cotton (Ed) Proceedings of a Symposium held at the Centre Interprofessionnel, Geneva, 8 March 1974, pp.111-117 (Elsevier, New York 1974).

Villarreal, H.; Exaire, J.E.; Rubio, V. and Davila, H. Effect of guanethidine and bretylium tosylate on systemic and renal hemodynamics in essential hypertension. American Journal of Cardiology 14: 633-640 (1964).

Villarreal, H.; Revollo, A.; Exaire, E. and Larrondo, F.: Effect of chlorothiazide on renal hemodynamics. Comparative study of acute administration in normotensive and hypertensive subjects. Circulation 26: 409-412 (1962).

Viveros, O.H.; Arqueros, L.; Connett, R.J. and Kirshner, N.: Mechanism of secretion from the adrenal medulla. IV. The fate of the storage vesicles following insulin and reserpine administration. Molecular Pharmacology 5: 69-82 (1969).

Vogt, M.: Catecholamines in brain. Pharmacological Reviews 11: 483-489 (1959).

Volle, R.L. and Koelle, G.B.: Ganglionic stimulating and blocking agents; in Goodman and Gilman (Eds) The Pharmacological Basis of Therapeutics, 5th ed., pp.565-574 (MacMillan, New York 1975).

Waal, H.J.: Propranolol-induced depression. British Medical Journal 2: 50 (1967).

Waal-Manning, H.J.: Hypertension: Which beta-blocker? Drugs 12: 412-441 (1976a).

Waal-Manning, H.J.: Metabolic effects of β-adrenoreceptor blockers. Drugs 11 (Suppl. 1): 121-126 (1976b).

Waal-Manning, H.J. and Simpson, F.O.: Paradoxical effect of pindolol. British Medical Journal 3: 155-156 (1975).

Wagner, J.: Pharmacokinetics and metabolism of hydralazine: Specific affinity for blood vessels. Experientia 29: 767 (1973).

Warren, D.J.: Beta-adrenergic receptor blockade and renal function. American Heart Journal 91: 265-266 (1976).

Warren, D.J.; Swainson, C.P. and Wright, N.: Deterioration in renal function after beta-blockade in patients with chronic renal failure and hypertension. British Medical Journal 2: 193-194 (1974).

Weil, M.H.; Barbour, B.H. and Chesne, R.B.: Alpha-methyldopa for the treatment of hypertension: Clinical and pharmacodynamic studies. Circulation 28: 165-174 (1963).

Weil, J.V. and Chidsey, C.A.: Plasma volume expansion resulting from interference with adrenergic function in normal man. Circulation 37: 54-61 (1968).

Weiner, N.: Regulation of norepinephrine biosynthesis. Annual Review of Pharmacology 10: 273-290 (1970).

Weiss, P.; Hersey, R.M.; Dujovne, C.A. and Bianchine, J.R.: The metabolism of amiloride hydrochloride in man. Clinical Pharmacology and Therapeutics 10: 401-406 (1969).

White, A.G.: Methyldopa and amitriptyline. Letter to the editor, Lancet 2: p441 (1965).

Wigand, M.E. and Heidland, A.: Ototoxic side effects of high doses of frusemide in patients with uraemia. Postgraduate Medical Journal (Suppl.): 54-56 (1971).

Wilkinson, E.L.; Backman, H. and Hecht, H.H.: Cardiovascular and renal adjustments to a hypotensive agent. Journal of Clinical Investigation 31: 872-879 (1952).

Wilson, D.J. and Vidt, D.G.: Control of severe hypertension with pulse doses of diazoxide. Clinical Pharmacology and Therapeutics 23: 135 (1978).

Wilson, W.R. and Okun, R.: The acute hemodynamic effects of diazoxide in man. Circulation 28: 89-93 (1963).

Wollam, G.L.; Bravo, E.L.; Dustan, H.P. and Tarazi, R.C.: Diuretic potency of combined thiazide and furosemide treatment in azotemic patients. Paper presented at the American College of Physicians Fifty-eighth annual session, Dallas, Texas, April, 1977.

Wollam, G.L.; Tarazi, R.C. and Bravo, E.L.: The acute hemodynamic effects and cardioselectivity of acebutolol: a comparison with practolol and propranolol. Clinical Pharmacology and Therapeutics 23: 136 (1978).

Wood, A.J.; Phelan, E.L. and Simpson, F.O.: Cardiovascular effects of prazosin in normotensive and genetically hypertensive rats. Clin. Exp. Pharmacol. Physiol. 2: 297-304 (1975).

Wood, A.J.; Bolli, P. and Simpson, F.O.: Prazosin in normal subjects: Plasma levels, blood pressure and heart rate. British Journal of Clinical Pharmacology 3: 199-201 (1976).

Wood, A.J.; Phelan, E.L. and Simpson, F.O.: Cardiovascular effects of prazosin in normotensive and genetically hypertensive rats. Clin. Exp. Pharmacol. Physiol. 2: 297-304 (1975).

Woods, J.W.; Pittman, A.W.; Pulliam, C.C.; Werk, E.E., Jr.; Waider, W. and Allen, C.A.: Renin profiling in hypertension and its use in treatment with propranolol and chlorthalidone. New England Journal of Medicine 294: 1137-1144 (1976).

Woosley, R.L. and Nies, A.S.: Guanethidine. New England Journal of Medicine 295: 1053-1056 (1976).

Woosley, R.L.; Walter, I.; Oates, J.A. and Nies, A.S.: Antagonism of the antihypertensive and sympathoplegic effects of guanethidine by ephedrine in man. Clinical Research 24: 259A (1976).

Worlledge, S.M.; Carstairs, K.C. and Dacie, J.V.: Autoimmune haemolytic anaemia associated with α-methyldopa therapy. Lancet 2: 135-139 (1966).

Zacest, R. and Koch-Weser, J.: Relation of hydralazine plasma concentration to dosage and hypotensive action. Clinical Pharmacology and Therapeutics 13: 420-425 (1972).

Zacest, R.; Gilmore, E. and Koch-Weser, J.: Treatment of essential hypertension with combined vasodilation and beta-adrenergic blockade. New England Journal of Medicine 286: 617-622 (1972).

Zacharias, F.J.; Cowen, K.J.; Prestt, J.; Vickers, J. and Wall, B.G.: Propranolol in hypertension. A study of long-term therapy, 1964-1970. American Heart Journal 83: 755-761 (1972).

Zarro, V.J.: The pharmacology of reserpine and guanethidine; in Onesti, Kim and Moyer (Eds) Hypertension: Mechanisms and Management, pp.283-287 (Grune and Stratton, New York 1973).

Chapter II

Metoprolol: A Review of its Pharmacological Properties and Therapeutic Efficacy in Hypertension

R.N. Brogden, R.C. Heel, T.M. Speight and G.S. Avery

1. Animal Pharmacodynamic Studies

In animal studies, metoprolol has been shown to possess β-adrenoceptor blocking activity, to exert a greater effect on β_1 than β_2 receptors, to be devoid of partial agonist activity, and to have only weak membrane stabilising activity. The pharmacological properties of metoprolol compared with those of some other β-adrenoceptor blocking drugs are shown in table I.

1.1 β-Adrenoceptor Blocking Effect

Metoprolol, in common with other β-adrenoceptor blocking drugs, antagonises the cardiovascular effects of isoprenaline in experimental animals (Ablad et al., 1973, 1974; Borg et al., 1975a). In anaesthetised cats with acute cardiac denervation, intravenous metoprolol 0.8 to 4mg/kg (Borg et al., 1975a) and 0.025 to 25.6mg/kg of practolol, H87/07[1], alprenolol, metoprolol and propranolol (Ablad et al., 1973) all produced dose dependent reduction in heart rate and contractile force. Metoprolol and practolol inhibited the chronotropic responses to intravenous noradrenaline, isoprenaline and adrenaline to a different degree in the order noradrenaline $>$

---

1 An experimental β_2-selective adrenoceptor blocking drug with intrinsic sympathomimetic activity.

Table I. Pharmacological properties. Some differences between various β-adrenoceptor blocking drugs

Drug	Beta blockade potency ratio (propranolol = 1)	Cardio-selectivity	Partial agonist	Membrane stabilising activity
Acebutolol	0.3	+	+	+
Alprenolol	1	0	+ +	+
Atenolol	1	+	0	0
Metoprolol	1	+	0	±
Oxprenolol	0.5-1	0	+ +	+
Pindolol	6	0	+ + +	+
Practolol	0.3	+	+ +	0
Propranolol	1	0	0	+ +
d-Propranolol	0.1	0	0	+ +
Sotalol	0.3	0	0	0
Timolol	6	0	±	0

isoprenaline > adrenaline, but the degree of inhibition with propranolol and alprenolol was more uniform, with the response to adrenaline being inhibited to the greatest extent (Ablad et al., 1974). The differentiated blockade pattern was also evident in the isolated cat heart preparation (Ablad et al., 1974) [see also section 3.3.1]. This suggests that metoprolol had little effect on the β-receptor mediated peripheral effect of adrenaline.

Propranolol and alprenolol were the most potent of the drugs tested at inhibiting the chronotropic response to isoprenaline, the ED_{50} being 4 to 6 times lower with propranolol and alprenolol (0.07 to 0.09mg/kg) than with the other three drugs (0.34 to 0.44mg/kg) [Ablad et al., 1973].

Whereas for propranolol and alprenolol, the ED_{50} for inhibition of the chronotropic response was the same for isoprenaline as for sympathetic nerve stimulation (vide supra), metoprolol, practolol and H87/07 inhibited the chronotropic response to electrical sympathetic nerve stimulation at lower doses than those required to inhibit the response to isoprenaline. ED_{50} values for these drugs

(0.05 to 0.08mg/kg) were slightly lower than for propranolol and alprenolol (0.10 to 0.13mg/kg).

1.2 Partial Agonist Activity

In reserpinised cats, intravenous metoprolol and propranolol did not influence heart rate or contractile force in cumulative doses of up to 0.85mg/kg, whereas practolol, alprenolol and H87/07 produced a dose dependent increase. An effect on contractile force was also observed with these three drugs when heart rate was kept constant by atrial pacing. These results indicated that metoprolol like propranolol is devoid of intrinsic β-adrenoceptor agonist activity (Ablad et al., 1973).

1.3 β-Adrenoceptor Selectivity

Metoprolol, like practolol, atenolol and H87/07 inhibits the cardiac effects of isoprenaline in cats at doses much lower than those required to inhibit the vasodilator response (Ablad et al., 1973; Lundgren, 1977). Similarly, the bronchodilator response to isoprenaline in guinea-pigs is blocked by doses of alprenolol and propranolol about 30 to 40 times less than those required for practolol and metoprolol (Ablad et al., 1973).

Propranolol and alprenolol inhibited the vasodilator response to intra-arterial isoprenaline at doses of 0.06 to 0.07mg/kg, closely similar to those required (0.07 to 0.09mg/kg) to inhibit the heart rate response. On the other hand, metoprolol and practolol inhibited the heart rate response to isoprenaline at doses of 0.34 to 0.44mg/kg, but 5 and 35mg/kg metoprolol and practolol respectively were required to inhibit the vasodilator response. On the basis of this experiment metoprolol is less 'cardioselective' than practolol or H87/07.

In beagle dogs (Ablad et al, 1974), the intravenous administration of metoprolol 0.4mg/kg before intravenous adrenaline infusion (0.5μg/kg/min) resulted in little change in mean aortic blood pressure (MABP) and a moderate increase in peripheral resistance (PR). This may have clinical application in situations where there is release of endogenous catecholamines. In contrast, propranolol 0.2mg/kg produced a marked increase in MABP due to greatly increased peripheral resistance. Thus, it appears that propranolol blocked the peripheral vasodilator effect of adrenaline thereby unmasking the α-adrenoceptor mediated vasoconstrictor effect (Ablad et al., 1974).

These findings suggest that metoprolol had little effect on the β-adrenoceptor mediated peripheral vasodilator effect of adrenaline and is more selective in its action than propranolol.

1.4 Antihypertensive Effect

Studies conducted in young spontaneously hypertensive rats indicated that metoprolol, like propranolol, largely prevented the increases in arterial blood pressure (Ljung et al., 1976; Ruskoaho and Karppanen, 1977; Weiss et al., 1974) and structural changes in resistance vessels seen in untreated age-matched controls (Weiss et al., 1974).

Treatment with metoprolol or propranolol 100mg/kg daily began at 2.5 months of age when mean arterial blood pressure in the spontaneously hypertensive rats was 135mm Hg compared with 115mm Hg in normotensive control rats. After 5.5 months of treatment with propranolol, mean arterial blood pressure was 138mm Hg compared with 175mm Hg in untreated age-matched spontaneously hypertensive controls. Similarly, after 5.5 months of treatment with metoprolol, mean arterial pressure was 137mm Hg compared with 175mm Hg in untreated controls.

Structural changes in resistance vessels were less marked in treated than in untreated rats and were similar to those seen in spontaneously hypertensive rats of 2.5 months of age. These findings suggest that further progression of hypertensive vascular changes was largely prevented. However, left ventricular hypertrophy had developed despite therapy and was only about 10% less than in untreated spontaneously hypertensive rats.

In contrast to findings subsequent to early treatment, Weiss et al. (1974) reported that treatment with propranolol begun after hypertension was 'established' (at 8 months of age), failed to lower the arterial pressure or prevent hypertensive vascular changes in resistance vessels, despite evidence of β-adrenoceptor blockade. However, 5 months oral treatment with 0.7mmol/kg daily metoprolol reduced blood pressure in 14 month spontaneously hypertensive rats compared with controls in a study conducted by Ljung et al. (1976).

1.5 Cardiovascular Haemodynamics in Dogs

Both propranolol and metoprolol at intravenous doses of 0.5mg/kg significantly reduced heart rate and cardiac output in beagle dogs pretreated with an anticholinergic agent to abolish cholinergic reflex adjustments (Ablad et al., 1974). Reduced cardiac output was accompanied by a corresponding increase in peripheral resistance so that mean aortic blood pressure was practically unchanged. Left ventricular end diastolic (EDD) and end systolic diameter (ESD) were increased after β-adrenoceptor blockade. These effects could probably be ascribed to negative cardiac chronotropic and inotropic actions resulting from inhibition of sympathetic activity in the heart. During exercise on a treadmill, heart rate and cardiac output were reduced compared with control values. There was no change in EDD, but ESD was increased. During atrial pacing at 220 beats per minute, stroke volume and maximum aortic blood flow acceleration were markedly decreased (Ablad et al., 1974).

1.6 Toxicology Studies

1.6.1 Acute Toxicity
In the mouse the LD_{50} of metoprolol was 69.4 to 79.9mg/kg intravenously and 2,460 (males) to 2,300mg/kg (females) orally. In the rat, LD_{50} values were 71.9 (male) to 74.3mg/kg (female) and 3,470 (female) to 4,670mg/kg (male) after intravenous and oral administration respectively (Bodin et al., 1975b).

1.6.2 Sub-acute Toxicity
In two beagle dogs, increasing doses of metoprolol from 40 to 100mg/kg for 6 days resulted in disturbances of balance, increased abdominal muscular tone, mydriasis and hyperaemia in visible mucous membranes 0.5 to 3 hours after administration, especially with high doses; one death occurred at a dose of 140mg/kg. In another 3 dogs, oral doses of 60mg/kg twice daily caused no clinical signs other than vomiting and increased salivation, but higher doses also caused incoordinated movements, tremor and ataxia. Doses of 120mg/kg twice daily proved fatal in a female dog, whilst a male dog died after 100mg/kg. No adverse clinical signs were noted following doses of 5, 20 and 40mg/kg daily for 1 month. Similarly, intravenous doses of 0.5 and 5mg/kg were well tolerated, with perivascular inflammatory changes at the site of injection being noted in control as well as in treated dogs.

In rats, oral doses of 10, 50 and 100mg/kg daily for 5 weeks and 200mg/kg daily for 3 weeks were without adverse clinical effects (Bodin et al., 1975b). The difference in the tolerated dosage levels in dogs and rats is no doubt related to the differences in bioavailability of metoprolol in the two species (section 2.1).

1.6.3 Chronic Toxicity
No adverse clinical effects in rats were associated with the oral administration of 10, 100 and 200mg/kg metoprolol daily for 6 months, and with 250mg/kg daily for 13 weeks. Similarly in beagle dogs, oral metoprolol 20 and 40mg/kg twice daily for 3 months and doses of 30mg/kg and 80mg/kg for 3 months, did not result in adverse clinical effects or any pathological changes attributable to the drug (Bodin et al., 1975a). No mention was made of ocular investigations or effects.

Carcinogenicity studies have been performed on rats and mice.

Groups of Sprague-Dawley rats, 50 males and 50 females in each group, were given 0, 50, 200 and 800mg/kg body weight a day. They were kept on a basal diet for another 26 weeks. No benign or malignant neoplasms of any type at any anatomical site in either sex in each of the 3 treatment groups occurred at a significantly increased incidence when compared with the incidence of identical types of neoplasm observed in the untreated control group.

Groups of Swiss albino mice, 50 males and 50 females in each group, were given 0, 75, 150 and 750mg/kg body weight a day for 78 weeks. The animals were kept on a basal diet for another 13 weeks. Numerous types of benign and malignant neo-plasm were discovered among the control mice and among the mice treated with metoprolol at all 3 dose levels. However, these tumours were distributed with equal frequency among all 4 groups and the conclusion was reached that metoprolol had no carcinogenic effect in this experiment (Malmfors, personal communication 1977).

1.7 Dysmorphology and Reproduction Studies

The size and weight of litters of Sprague-Dawley female rats given oral metoprolol 10, 50 and 200mg/kg on days 6 to 15 of gestation were not adversely affected by the drug. Skeletal and visceral examination did not reveal abnormalities attributable to the drug. In New Zealand white rabbits given metoprolol 5, 12.5 and 25mg/kg daily on days 6 to 18 of gestation, there was a slight reduction in litter size and a slight increase in fetal loss at the highest dose level. Fetal abnormalities did not appear to be influenced by the drug (Bodin et al., 1975b). Oral metoprolol 10, 50 and 200mg/kg was without adverse effect on duration of gestation, labour, delivery or lactation in Sprague-Dawley rats treated from day 15 of gestation to 21 days post partum. Likewise, litter size, pup weight at birth and at 14 and 21 days post partum, cumulative fetal loss and incidence of gross malformations were not adversely affected by metoprolol at the dosages used (Bodin et al., 1975b).

A significant reduction in the number of viable newborn Charles River rats and an increase in the frequency of stillbirths was noted only following oral administra-tion of metoprolol 500mg/kg daily to males and females prior to mating and during mating, and to females throughout gestation and lactation periods. Postnatal survival of pups was decreased when compared with controls in the 500 and 50mg/kg groups, but differences were not statistically significant for the low dose group on 50mg/kg daily. The postnatal growth of surviving pups was not impaired (Bodin et al., 1975b).

2. Animal Pharmacokinetic Studies

2.1 Absorption

Metoprolol appears to be almost completely absorbed from the gastrointestinal tract, as evidenced by the high urinary recovery following the oral administration of 100mg/kg daily to rats and 20mg/kg to dogs, the relative independence of route of administration and low faecal levels of radioactivity following administration of tri-tium-labelled drug (Borg et al., 1975b).

In the rat, about 95% of an oral dose was eliminated during the first pass through the liver (i.e. bioavailability is about 5%) whilst in the dog bioavailability is about 20 to 40% (Borg et al., 1975a,b) after oral doses of 0.4 to 2mg/kg, and is similar to that in man (section 4.1).

2.2 Half-life

The plasma half-life as calculated from the linear part of the bi-exponential plasma concentration versus time curve, was 1.3 to 1.7 hours in conscious beagle dogs, irrespective of the route of administration, 1.3 hours in the cat and 0.6 to 0.74 hours in the untreated and pretreated rat respectively (Borg et al., 1975a,b).

2.3 Distribution

Studies with tritium-labelled metoprolol indicate that in the mouse and the rat, the tissue distribution of the drug is typical of that of a moderately lipophilic basic drug. It is similar to propranolol except that there is less in the brain and lung. After intravenous administration, highest levels of radioactivity due to unchanged drug were found in lungs and kidneys. In the liver, the radioactivity was due almost entirely to metabolites (Bodin et al., 1975a). The apparent volume of distribution was 5.52 ± 0.64L/kg in the cat and 3.09 to 3.61L/kg in the dog (Borg et al., 1975a).

2.4 Metabolism

In the dog and rat, as in man (section 4.4), metoprolol is largely metabolised. Borg et al. (1975c) detected 3 metabolites by gas chromatography and mass spectrometry, whilst Arfwidsson et al. (1976) reported a further 4 urinary metabolites in the rat, *in vitro* and *in vivo*. The relative percentage of the 3 main metabolites in the rat was not altered significantly by pretreatment with phenobarbitone or with metoprolol (Arfwidsson et al., 1976). 2 of the 3 metabolites defined by Borg et al. (1975c) were without effect on the cardiovascular responses to isoprenaline, whilst the third metabolite was less active and had a lower acute toxicity than metoprolol.

3. Human Pharmacodynamic Studies

3.1 Effect on Heart Rate and Cardiac Output

Acute or chronic administration of metoprolol to normal subjects or hypertensive patients results in a reduction in heart rate and cardiac output which appears to be related to the dose of the drug. Stroke volume is unchanged.

In 14 female hypertensive patients who had been receiving treatment with metoprolol 150 to 240mg daily for up to 13 months, a single 50 or 80mg dose given

1 to 4 weeks after cessation of long term treatment, caused a reduction in resting heart rate of 13 and 15bpm respectively (Bengtsson et al., 1975). During chronic administration, a 50mg dose reduced the resting heart rate by 8bpm whilst an 80mg dose caused a reduction of 11bpm. The effect was still significant 6 hours after a dose (Bengtsson et al., 1975). Similarly, Hansson et al. (1977a) noted a reduction of 13 and 19bpm in the supine and standing heart rate (resting) respectively, during chronic administration of metoprolol 150 to 450mg daily to 9 male patients with essential hypertension. The increase in heart rate caused by maximal or submaximal exercise was significantly reduced by chronic metoprolol administration (Hansson et al., 1977a,b). A dose related reduction in exercise tachycardia after oral administration of 20, 50 and 100mg or intravenous administration of 5, 10, 15 and 20mg was noted by Johnsson (1975a). For identical response, the ratio between oral and intravenous doses was about 2.5:1 (see also section 4.1). The degree of β-adrenoceptor blockade as reflected in the reduction in exercise tachycardia and resting pulse rate was found by von Bahr et al. (1976) to be correlated with the mean steady-state plasma concentration.

In a comparison of single doses of metoprolol and propranolol in 6 subjects (Johnsson et al. 1975b), exercise-induced increase in heart rate was reduced to about the same extent by 40mg orally of either drug. The effect of 80mg metoprolol was significantly greater than that of the 40mg dose but not significantly different from that of 40mg propranolol. Metoprolol 100 and 200mg daily reduced exercise-induced increase in heart rate to a similar extent as atenolol 100 and 200mg in 7 hypertensive subjects (Comerford and Besterman, 1977).

Intravenous metoprolol 0.15mg/kg significantly reduced cardiac output at rest (17%) and during exercise (22%) in volunteers (Stenberg et al., 1975) and in hypertensive patients (Sannerstedt and Wasir, 1977). The reduction in cardiac output was considered to be due mainly to reduced heart rate (13 to 18%), stroke volume being unchanged at rest and only slightly reduced during exercise (Sannerstedt and Wasir, 1977; Stenberg et al., 1975). A slightly greater reduction in heart rate (22% at rest, 20% exercise) and in cardiac output (22% at rest, 17% exercise) was reported by Lund-Johansen and Ohm (1977) during 1 year's treatment with metoprolol 50 to 250mg daily alone in 12 men with previously untreated mild essential hypertension.

In a comparison of the long term haemodynamic effects of alprenolol (400 to 800mg daily), atenolol (100 to 200mg), timolol (10 to 20mg) and metoprolol (50 to 300mg), all drugs produced a comparable reduction in cardiac output but the fall in heart rate was most pronounced with atenolol and timolol (Lund-Johansen and Ohm, 1976).

3.2 Effect on Blood Pressure

Single doses of metoprolol given orally or intravenously to normal subjects or hypertensive patients rapidly lower systolic blood pressure. Although diastolic

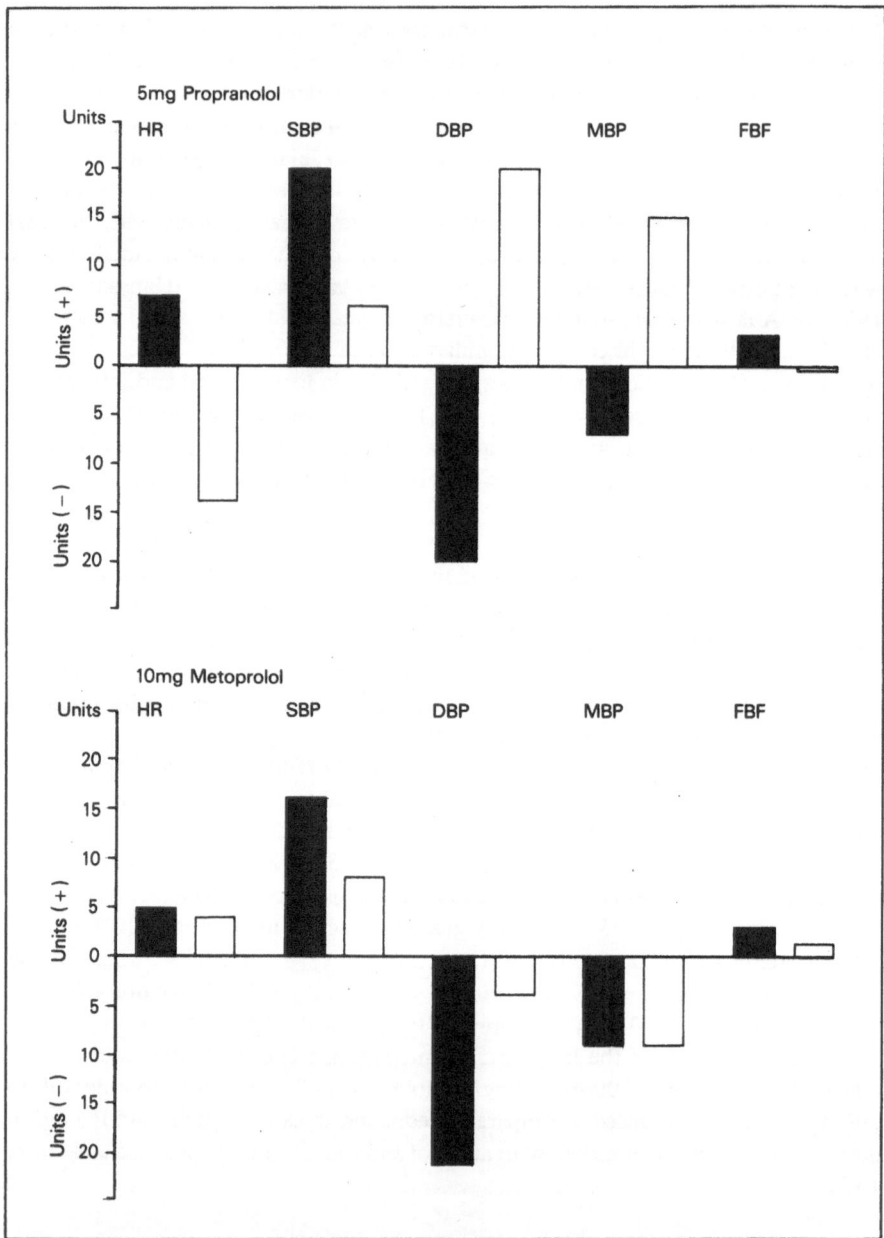

Fig. 1. Effect of adrenaline infusion (0.1µg/kg/min) on heart rate (HR), systolic blood pressure (SBP), diastolic blood pressure (DBP), mean blood pressure (MBP) and forearm blood flow (FBF), before ■ and after □ intravenous administration of propranolol or metoprolol (after Johnsson, 1975a).

pressure was not reduced by a single dose it was significantly reduced by 150 to 450mg daily for 3 to 4 weeks (Ekelund et al., 1976; Hansson et al., 1977a).

Administration of a single 80mg oral dose of metoprolol to patients who had been treated continuously with metoprolol up to 1 to 4 weeks before the experiment, resulted in a significant lowering of systolic but not diastolic blood pressure (Bengtsson et al., 1975). The effect was apparent within 15 minutes of ingestion, was maximal at 2 hours and lasted for at least 6 hours. A similar finding was reported by Nyberg (1976). The oral administration of 100mg metoprolol significantly lowered systolic but not diastolic blood pressure in normal subjects. The effect of a 50mg dose was less pronounced. The effect on blood pressure was not significantly correlated with the plasma concentration, although there was a trend towards such a relationship. Johnsson et al. (1975a) reported that the hypotensive effect of oral and intravenous metoprolol on the systolic blood pressure during exercise was related to the dose in 5 healthy subjects given 20, 50 and 100mg orally, and 5, 10, 15 and 20mg intravenously.

No significant difference between the effects of 40 and 80mg metoprolol and 40mg propranolol on exercise-induced increase in blood pressure could be detected by Johnsson et al. (1975b); nor between 100 and 200mg metoprolol and 100 and 200mg atenolol by Comerford and Besterman (1977). Metoprolol 450mg daily significantly reduced systolic blood pressure during maximal work, but diastolic pressure was not reduced (Hansson et al., 1977a).

Increases in indirectly measured blood pressure resulting from isometric exercise were not significantly lowered by metoprolol, although a fall in blood pressure was noted on direct measurement (Hunyor and Nyberg, 1978).

3.3 β-Adrenoceptor Selectivity

3.3.1 Effect on Haemodynamic Response to Sympathomimetic Agents

As in animals (section 1.3), metoprolol and propranolol differ considerably in their effects on the haemodynamic response to infused adrenaline (Johnson, 1975a; van Herwaarden et al., 1977) or isoprenaline (Johnsson et al., 1975b) [fig. 1].

Although the effect of 40mg doses of metoprolol and propranolol on exercise-induced increase in heart rate is similar (section 3.1), their effect on the isoprenaline-induced increase in heart rate differed considerably. The increase in heart rate induced by isoprenaline was reduced more by 40mg oral propranolol (from 30 ± 6 to 2 ± 1) 90 minutes after drug ingestion than by either 40mg (from 31 ± 9 to 28 ± 6) or 80mg (36 ± 9 to 19 ± 5) of metoprolol. Similar results were obtained after intravenous propranolol (0.06mg/kg) and metoprolol (0.12mg/kg) [Johnsson et al., 1975c].

Adrenaline causes vasodilatation in muscle by activation of β2-adrenoceptors. After a single intravenous dose of propranolol this vasodilating action is lost, and

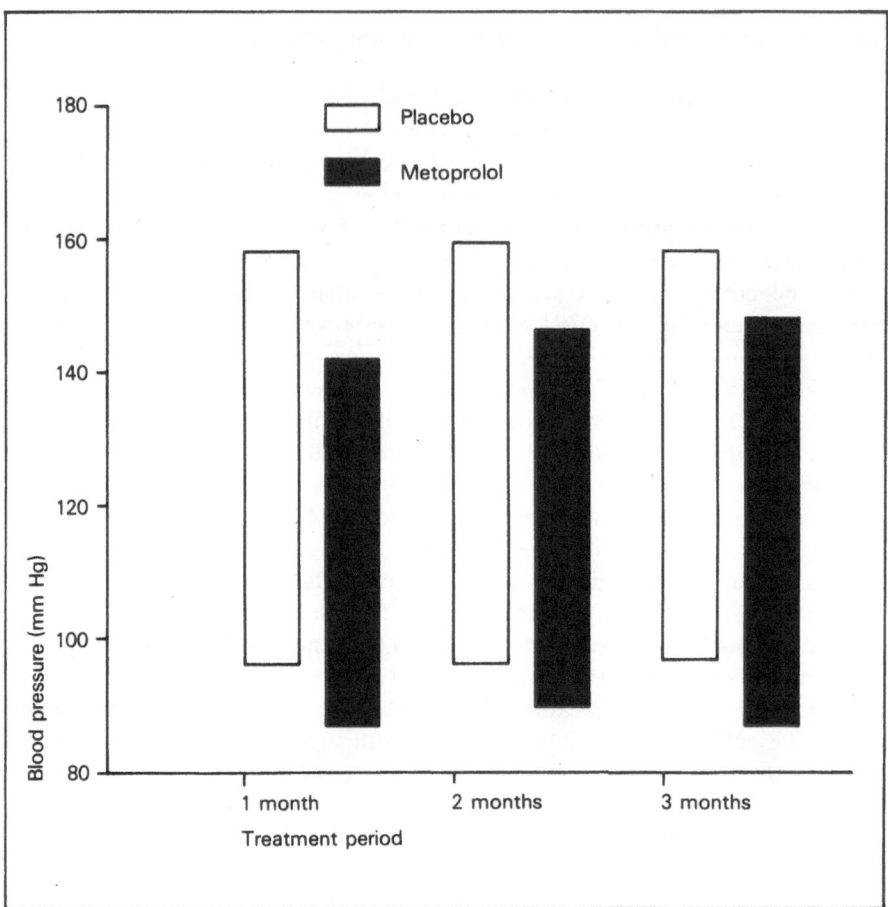

Fig. 2. Mean values for supine systolic and diastolic blood pressure during a double-blind comparison of metoprolol and placebo in patients with mild to moderate essential hypertension receiving chlorthalidone 25mg daily (after Jaattela and Pyorala, 1976).

there is vasoconstriction, an increase in peripheral vascular resistance and a rise in blood pressure, presumably as a result of α-adrenoceptor stimulation. After a single intravenous dose of metoprolol, the vasodilating action of adrenaline (0.1 μg/kg/min) is largely preserved (fig. 1) [van Herwaarden et al., 1977; Johnsson, 1975a].

The difference in the interaction of the two β-adrenoceptor blocking drugs with adrenaline is interpreted as being the result of a much less pronounced effect of metoprolol on the adrenergic β_2-receptors compared with propranolol. Further evidence of the selectivity of metoprolol is illustrated by its minimal effect on lung function (section 3.3.2).

3.3.2 Effect on Lung Function and Response to β_2-Adrenoceptor Stimulants

In asthmatic patients not experiencing an exacerbation of their asthma, single (Benson et al., 1977; Thiringer and Svedmyr, 1976; Singh et al., 1976) or repeated oral (Tivenius, 1976) [50 to 100mg] or single intravenous doses (0.12mg/kg; 8mg) of metoprolol (Johnsson et al., 1975c; Skinner et al., 1976) generally cause some reduction in basal FEV_1 (Benson et al., 1977; Johnsson et al., 1975c; Skinner et al., 1976; Tivenius, 1976; Thiringer and Svedmyr, 1976), FVC (Skinner et al., 1976) and specific airways resistance (Singh et al., 1976). This effect is less than that produced by equiactive β-blocking doses of propranolol (table II). Unlike propranolol however, metoprolol does not significantly inhibit the bronchodilatation induced by infused isoprenaline (Johnsson et al., 1975c; Thiringer and Svedmyer, 1976), or by inhaled isoprenaline (Benson et al., 1977; Tivenius, 1976).

In one study (Skinner et al., 1976), there was no significant difference between the effect on the airways of intravenous metoprolol 8mg and placebo on the basis of effect on specific airways conductance, although metoprolol had a greater effect than placebo on FEV_1 and FVC. The bronchoconstriction was readily reversed by salbutamol. However, in a study of atenolol, metoprolol, acebutolol, pindolol, oxprenolol and propranolol in patients with stable reversible obstructive airways disease (Benson et al., 1977), only atenolol permitted a bronchodilator response to isoprenaline that did not differ significantly from that with placebo. The response to isoprenaline after metoprolol was greater than after propranolol or oxprenolol. Studies were performed in patients who had been shown to experience a 20% or greater fall in FEV_1 with at least one of the β-adrenoceptor blocking drugs.

The effects on FEV_1 of 17 days treatment with oral metoprolol (100mg and 200mg daily) and practolol (200 and 400mg daily) in 17 hypertensive patients with asthma, which in 13 required regular steroid therapy, and who were receiving optimum β_2-adrenoceptor-stimulant therapy with terbutaline, were studied by Formgren (1976). In the low dose period, there was no difference in FEV_1 between placebo and either drug or between the active drugs. At the higher doses, there was a reduction in FEV_1 with both drugs, but no significant difference between the drugs. The same 4 patients experienced exacerbation of their asthma during treatment with the higher dose of each drug. Horvath et al. (1977) reported that a significant fall in maximal mid-expiratory flow rate (MMFR) occurred in hypertensive patients (non-asthmatic) receiving either propranolol 320mg or metoprolol 400mg for 2 weeks. However, MMFR fell significantly in 7 of 10 patients whilst on propranolol and in 2 of these patients whilst receiving metoprolol. It should be stressed that concomitant optimum therapy with β_2-adrenoceptor stimulants is mandatory in any asthmatic patients in whom treatment with 'cardioselective' drugs is contemplated. However, even in these circumstances, exacerbation of asthma is likely with the doses of β_1-selective adrenoceptor blocking drugs usually used in the treatment of hypertension.

Table II. Changes in mean basal FEV$_1$, FVC and specific airways resistance (SRaw) and in isoprenaline induced bronchodilatation in asthmatic patients given metoprolol, propranolol, practolol and placebo

Author	Test	Placebo	Metoprolol (dose)	Propranolol (dose)	Practolol (dose)
Johnsson			(0.12mg/kg iv)	(0.06mg/kg iv)	—
et al. (1975c)	FEV$_1$ (b)[1]	-0.04L	-0.12L	-0.20L	
	FVC (b)	-0.08L	-0.06L	-0.34L	—
	FEV$_1$ (i)[2]	+ 0.56L	+ 0.50L	+ 0.10L	—
Singh	SRaw		(100mg)	(80mg)	(250mg)
et al. (1976)		+ 10.45	+ 30.54	+ 34.12	+ 32.93
Skinner			(8mg iv)	(5mg iv)	
et al. (1976)	FEV$_1$ (b)	-0.06L	-0.28L	-0.44L	
	FVC (b)	-0.09L	-0.37L	-0.55L	
Tivenius (1976)			(50mg tid)	(40mg tid)	
	FEV$_1$ (i)	+ 0.17L	+ 0.19L	+ 0.11L	
	FVC (i)	+ 0.30L	+ 0.29L	+ 0.22L	
Thiringer and			(50mg; 100mg)	(40mg)	(200mg)
Svedmyr (1977)	FEV$_1$ (b)	-0.06L	-0.18L	-0.28L	-0.08L
	FEV$_1$ (i)	+ 0.48L	+ 0.50L;0.48L	+ 0.10L	+ 0.44L

1   FEV$_1$ (b) = basal forced expiratory volume in one second. FVC (b) — basal forced vital capacity.

2   FEV$_1$ (i) = forced expiratory volume in one second after administration of isoprenaline. FVC (i) = forced vital capacity after administration of isoprenaline.

3.4 Effect on Plasma Renin Activity

Metoprolol, given continuously (von Bahr et al., 1976; Pfisterer et al., 1976) or in single doses (Attman et al., 1975), reduces plasma renin activity (PRA) in hypertensive patients and in normal subjects. It may also reduce PRA in hypertensive patients previously treated with pindolol, practolol or oxprenolol (Waal-Manning, 1976a).

In 7 volunteers (Attman et al., 1975), the effect on frusemide-stimulated plasma renin activity of 40mg oral metoprolol and propranolol was compared with that of placebo. PRA increased by 0.59 ± 0.18ng/ml/h after frusemide and placebo, but the corresponding increase was statistically significantly less after propranolol (0.16 ± 0.06) or metoprolol (0.24 ± 0.08ng/ml/h).

Chronic administration of metoprolol 300mg daily reduced both standing (2.6 $\pm$ 0.3 to 0.7 $\pm$ 0.1ng/ml/h) and supine (1.8 $\pm$ 0.2 to 0.6 $\pm$ 0.1ng/ml/h) PRA in hypertensive patients (von Bahr et al., 1976). The rise in PRA after 4 hours in the standing position was significant during placebo but not during metoprolol treatment. In another study (Pfisterer et al., 1976), metoprolol and propranolol 150mg daily for 4 weeks resulted in comparable falls in PRA in hypertensive patients. In hypertensive patients who had been treated with either practolol, pindolol or oxprenolol, substitution of metoprolol resulted in a trend towards a decrease in PRA (Waal-Manning, 1976a). This change (2.37 to 1.95ng/ml/h) became significant when patients taking the other three β-adrenoceptor blocking drugs were considered together. Like other investigators, Waal-Manning (1976a) found that metoprolol produced a significant decrease in PRA in hypertensive patients not previously treated with a β-adrenoceptor blocking agent.

3.5 Metabolic Effects

3.5.1 Serum Glucose and Insulin Levels
It is thought that the adrenergic receptor which modulates insulin secretion may be a β_2-receptor (Loubatieres et al., 1971), which might be affected to a lesser degree by a β_1-adrenoceptor selective blocking drug such as metoprolol than by a non-selective drug such as propranolol.

Studies with metoprolol in healthy volunteers (Davidson et al., 1977; Newman, 1976) and in hypertensive patients (Hansson et al., 1977b) have reported differing findings. Whereas Newman (1976) reported that oral metoprolol 100mg daily for 2 days delayed the return to normoglycaemia subsequent to insulin induced hypoglycaemia in 11 fasting volunteers, Davidson et al. (1977) found a normal response following insulin hypoglycaemia in 5 fasted volunteers given intravenous metoprolol 20mg followed by an infusion of 6mg per hour. In both of these studies, an equivalent dosage of propranolol caused a delayed return to normal blood glucose levels. In 9 hypertensive males treated with metoprolol 150 to 450mg daily for 4 to 17 weeks (Hansson et al., 1977b), the return to normal blood glucose after insulin was not significantly different from that during placebo.

No evidence of decreased insulin production in response to an oral or intravenous glucose load, nor changes in fasting levels of blood glucose or plasma insulin were noted by Ekberg and Hansson (1977) in hypertensive patients treated with metoprolol 150 to 450mg daily for 3 months.

In the only study so far in mildly diabetic patients, Waal-Manning (1976a) observed that substitution of metoprolol for previous therapy with propranolol (2 patients), pindolol (7), alprenolol (1) or oxprenolol (6), tended to increase glucose tolerance at 1 and 6 months and resulted in a significant increase in serum insulin levels after glucose. Further suitably designed studies are required to determine the effects and any advantages of metoprolol in patients with diabetes mellitus.

Table III. Some pharmacokinetic values of metoprolol and other commonly used β-adrenoceptor blocking drugs

Drug	Extent of absorption (% of dose)	Bioavailability (% of dose)	Distribution volume (L/kg)	Protein binding (%)	Elimination T$_{1/2}$(h)	Urinary recovery (% of dose)		Active metabolites of clinical importance
						unchanged	total	
Alprenolol	> 90	≈ 10	3.3	85	2-3	< 1	> 90	Yes
Metoprolol	> 95	≈ 40-50[1]	5.6	12	3-4	≈ 3	> 95	No
Oxprenolol	70-95	24-60			1-2		70-95	
Pindolol	> 90	≈ 100	2.0	57[1]	3-4	≈ 40	> 90	No
Practolol	> 95	≈ 100	1.6	32[2]	5-13	> 90	> 90	No
Propranolol	> 90	≈ 30	3.6	93	2-3	< 1	> 90	Yes

1 Bioavailability increases to 50% as dosage is increased to 100mg.
2 Percentage of a dose bound to human serum albumin.

3.5.2 Plasma Lipids and Catecholamines

Although a significant rise in fasting trigylcerides during metoprolol therapy has been reported by some investigators (Waal-Manning, 1976a; Hua, personal communication), others have found no consistent changes (Bengtsson, 1976a, Hansson et al., 1977b; Harms et al., 1978; Nilsson et al., 1977).

No consistent changes have been seen in basal catecholamine or fasting free fatty acid levels (FFA) in hypertensive patients receiving metoprolol 150 to 450mg daily (Hansson et al., 1977b; Nilsson et al., 1977; Newman, personal communication), whereas fasting FFA levels were reduced and FFA mobilisation inhibited by propranolol and acebutolol (Newman, personal communication). An increase in plasma adrenaline response to insulin hypoglycaemia during metoprolol, gréater than before treatment, was noted by Hansson et al. (1977b) and by Hokfelt et al. (1978) who also noted an increase in plasma levels of growth hormone and a slight increase in plasma cortisol. During submaximal work, plasma adrenaline was not altered by metoprolol whereas plasma noradrenaline was enhanced. The increase in plasma glycerol due to work was inhibited by metoprolol therapy (150 to 450mg daily) [Nilsson et al., 1977].

Fasting plasma triglyceride levels increased significantly (102 to 137mg/ 100ml) after 3 months of therapy with metoprolol both in patients (14) who had not

previously been treated with β-adrenoceptor blocking drugs and in 21 patients in
whom metoprolol was substituted for other β-adrenoceptor blocking drugs (increase
from 136 to 194mg/100ml) [Waal-Manning, 1976a].

4. Pharmacokinetic Studies in Man

Metoprolol is readily and rapidly absorbed after oral administration and is
rapidly distributed to body tissues. Plasma levels vary considerably between individuals, probably because of significant hepatic 'first-pass elimination' which results
in 50% of the administered oral dose reaching the systemic circulation. Metoprolol is
only slightly bound to human serum protein, namely albumin, which is reflected in
its large volume of distribution. The elimination half-life of metoprolol is about 3 to 4
hours in most patients (range 2.5 to 7.5h) and is independent of dose and duration of
therapy. The drug undergoes extensive biotransformation, and is excreted principally
via the kidneys, only about 3% being excreted as the unchanged drug after oral administration and about 10% after intravenous administration. The metabolites have
no clinically important activity. Comparison of the pharmacokinetic properties of
metoprolol with those of other β-adrenoceptor blocking drugs is given in table III.

4.1 Absorption

Studies with oral and intravenous tritiated metoprolol indicate that the drug is
rapidly and completely absorbed (Regardh et al., 1974, 1975). Absorption appears to
take place over a wide part of the intestine as radioactive doses given as ordinary or
slow-release tablets of varying dissolution rates were almost completely recovered in
the urine (Regardh et al., 1975). The estimated half-life of the absorption process is
about 10 to 12 minutes (Regardh et al., 1974; Johnsson and Regardh, 1976) when
metoprolol is administered as a weakly acidic solution. The rate of absorption is influenced by the dissolution rate of the oral preparation, peak plasma levels being attained
1.5h after ordinary tablets and 4h after slow-release tablets. Plama drug concentrations after intravenous administration are higher than after an oral dose (Johnsson et
al., 1975a) and for an identical reduction in exercise heart rate the ratio between oral
and intravenous doses is about 2.5 (Johnsson et al., 1975a).

About 40% of an oral dose of 5mg metoprolol is available to the systemic circulation (Regardh et al., 1974), although bioavailability increases to about 50% as
the dose is increased to 100mg (Johnsson et al., 1975a).

Plasma metoprolol levels vary considerably between individuals and reach a
peak at about 1.5h after oral administration (Bengtsson et al., 1975; Regardh et al.,
1975). After administration of single doses of 50mg and 80mg to 14 hypertensive
patients, peak plasma levels ranged from 35 to 125ng/ml and 48 to 184ng/ml respectively. During long term treatment with metoprolol, plasma levels were 33 to

246ng/ml and 106 to 208ng/ml respectively after doses of 50 and 80mg (Bengtsson et al., 1975). A similar rise in steady-state compared with single dose plasma levels was reported by Regardh et al. (1975) in 6 healthy volunteers in whom maximum plasma concentrations ranged from 46 to 270ng/ml after single 100mg doses given in ordinary tablet form. Steady-state levels ranged from 93 to 394ng/ml. Ingestion of slow-release tablets resulted in lower peak plasma levels of metoprolol which were attained at about 4 hours. Although the mean area under the plasma concentration-time curve tended to be greater after the ordinary tablet the difference was not statistically significant (Regardh et al., 1975).

Direct proportionality between plasma concentration and dose was obtained with intravenous doses above 10mg and oral doses above 50mg, but the ratio of the increase with dosage was higher at lower dosage levels. The increased bioavailability with increasing doses suggests the presence of some saturable disposition process of low capacity, especially after oral administration (Johnsson et al., 1975a).

A study by Kendall et al. (1977) investigated plasma concentrations of metoprolol in young volunteers, elderly but otherwise fit subjects and hypertensive patients. Each group consisted of 6 males and 2 females; the elderly group were all over 62 years of age. All subjects received a single 100mg oral dose of metoprolol. The plasma concentration-time profile did not differ between the young volunteers and hypertensive subjects, there being no statistically significant difference in the mean curve or area under the plasma concentration-time curve; this confirms the findings of Bengtsson et al. (1975) who studied smaller doses over a 6-hour period.

Although there was no statistically significant difference in the area under the curve between the elderly group and the young or hypertensive groups, the interindividual variations in plasma concentration in the elderly group were much more marked and the mean peak concentrations tended to be higher (about 1.5 times) and to occur later (4 cf 2h), with plasma concentrations at 24 hours in the elderly tending to be higher than the concentration at 12 hours in the young volunteers.

Other studies have also pointed to the much greater interindividual variability in peak plasma concentrations as well as in elimination half-life in the elderly compared with young subjects (section 4.3). Further studies are necessary to determine whether a reduction in dosage or dose frequency is appropriate in some elderly patients.

4.2 Distribution

Metoprolol reaches concentrations in the erythrocytes about 20% higher than in the plasma after administration of therapeutic doses (Regardh et al., 1974). Wood (1977) reported a concentration of metoprolol of 267ng/ml in the cerebrospinal fluid when the corresponding concentration in the plasma of a patient receiving 50mg 3 times daily was 341ng/ml. Peak concentrations of metoprolol in saliva are considerably higher than those in plasma (Dawes et al., 1978).

Metoprolol has a high volume of distribution of 5.6L/kg (Regardh et al., 1974) which appears to be due mainly to the low degree of binding to human plasma proteins (Johansson et al., 1974). Metoprolol is only about 11% bound to human serum protein and appears to be bound solely to serum albumin (Appelgren et al., 1974; Johansson et al., 1974). In the same study, alprenolol was found to be 85% bound to serum proteins. After oral administration of metoprolol, the plasma concentration curves do not show any clearcut distribution phase (α-phase), but this phase is clearly apparent after an intravenous dose (Regardh et al., 1974) when the half-life of the distribution phase is about 12 minutes.

4.3 Metabolism and Excretion

Only about 3% of an oral dose and 10% of an intravenous dose of metoprolol is recovered in the urine as unchanged drug (Regardh et al., 1974). Metoprolol is extensively metabolised in the liver. The hydroxy derivative of metoprolol which accounts for about 10% of the urinary activity, has some β-adrenoceptor blocking activity, but this appears to be of no clinical significance (Johnsson and Regardh, 1976). Three main metabolites of metoprolol have been isolated in man (Borg et al., 1975c) as well as in the rat and the dog. These three metabolites account for 85% of the total urinary excretion in man (Borg et al., 1975c). The main metabolite of metoprolol in man, as well as in the dog and rat, is an amino acid formed by 0-demethylation and oxidation (Borg et al., 1975c).

In healthy subjects, the renal clearance is 109ml/min for the unchanged drug and 120ml/min for the metabolites (Regardh et al., 1974). This value indicates that glomerular filtration mainly determines the excretion of metoprolol, although the existence of tubular secretion and reabsorption of about equal efficacy cannot be disregarded (Regardh et al., 1974).

About 95% of an oral or intravenous dose of metoprolol is recovered in the urine over a period of 72 hours. Whereas the elimination half-life of the total metabolites after oral administration is about 3 hours, that after an intravenous dose is about 5 hours, indicating that the route of administration might influence the metabolic pathways of metoprolol.

The elimination half-life of metoprolol in most patients is about 3 to 4 hours (range 2.5 to 7.5) and is independent of dose. The elimination half-life (3.7 hours) in elderly patients (Lundborg and Steen, 1975) is about the same as in younger healthy volunteers (e.g. Johnsson et al., 1975a; Regardh et al., 1975). However, the interindividual variation in peak plasma levels and elimination half-lives seemed to be more pronounced in the elderly patients.

The finding that the elimination half-life is almost the same after single doses or long term administration indicates that metoprolol does not inhibit or induce its own metabolism (Bengtsson et al., 1975). However, there is some cumulation after repeated doses, mean plasma levels after a morning dose on long term therapy being 45% higher than those after a single dose (Bengtsson et al., 1975).

4.4 Plasma Concentration and Clinical Effects

A significant relationship between the effect of metoprolol on heart rate and blood pressure during exercise and the logarithm of plasma drug concentration was reported by Regardh et al. (1975), but the relationship between plasma concentration and percentage reduction of systolic blood pressure in hypertensive patients was not significant in the study of Bengtsson et al. (1975). Similarly, there was no correlation between the plasma concentration and the change in diastolic blood pressure after 4 months of therapy with metoprolol in 24 hypertensive patients studied by Edvardsson et al. (1976) [cited in Johnsson and Regardh, 1976]. A direct correlation between plasma metoprolol and reduction in exercise tachycardia in patients with angina pectoris was noted by Keyrilainen and Uusitalo (1975).

Because of the wide individual variation in plasma concentrations (section 4.1), their determination in hypertensive patients is of limited value for the adjustment of the dose in routine therapy. Monitoring of plasma levels may however prove valuable in selected cases, such as those with impaired liver or renal function or in the elderly.

5. Therapeutic Trials

Controlled therapeutic trials in patients with essential hypertension have shown metoprolol to be an effective β-adrenoceptor blocking drug in this disease. In all placebo-controlled studies, metoprolol has been superior to placebo and in comparative studies, the effects of metoprolol have been statistically indistinguishable from those of equivalent β-blocking doses of propranolol. Trials comparing several β-adrenoceptor blocking drugs in moderate essential hypertension have shown that antihypertensive activity of individually titrated doses of metoprolol to be similar to that of the other β-adrenoceptor blocking drugs at dosages producing an equivalent degree of β-blockade.

5.1 Comparison with Placebo

Double-blind studies comparing metoprolol with placebo in patients with mild to moderate essential hypertension have shown that metoprolol is superior to placebo under controlled conditions. A fixed dose of metoprolol was used in the study of Bengtsson (1976a) whilst Jaattela and Pyorala (1976) and Waal-Manning (1976b) used individually titrated doses of the β-adrenoceptor blocking drug.

In a well designed study in 23 patients with mild to moderate essential hypertension receiving chlorthalidone 25mg daily, Jaattela and Pyorala (1976) compared the

effects of titrated doses of metoprolol with those of an equal number of placebo
tablets. During a 3-month pretrial period patients whose diastolic blood pressure remained above 95mm Hg despite 2 months of treatment with chlorthalidone 25mg
daily, received metoprolol at a dosage which reduced their blood pressure to ≤95mm
Hg. Most patients (17/23) received 150 to 225mg of metoprolol daily in 3 divided
doses, the arbitrarily chosen maximum dose of metoprolol being 300mg daily. By the
third week of the titration period, supine diastolic blood pressure was below 95mm
Hg in 19 patients.

  During the 6-month trial period, patients received either metoprolol or placebo
in addition to chlorthalidone for 3 months, then the alternative preparation for the remaining 3 months. Mean values for diastolic and systolic blood pressure in the supine
and standing position were significantly lower during metoprolol than placebo (fig.
3). A supine diastolic blood pressure of <95mm Hg was achieved in 22 of 23
patients at the end of the metoprolol period and in 12 of the 23 patients at the end of
the placebo period. Dizziness and tiredness occurred more frequently during

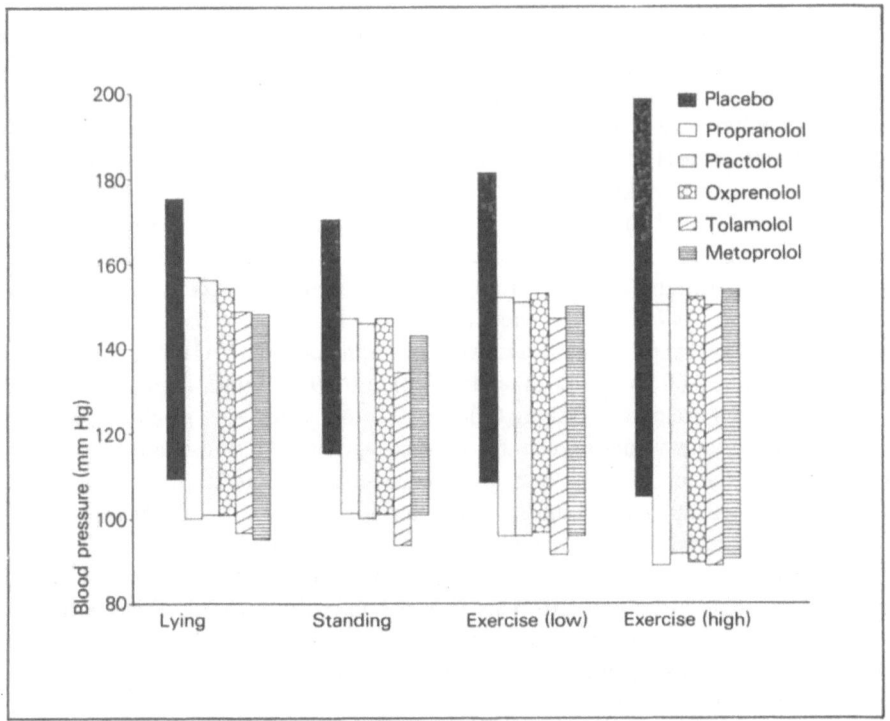

Fig. 3. Blood pressure recordings after 8 weeks of treatment with 5 different β-adrenoceptor
blocking drugs in a placebo controlled trial in 25 patients with uncomplicated essential hypertension
(after Davidson et al., 1976).

metoprolol than during placebo administration, but these effects appeared to diminish with time. In no case did side effects interfere with normal daily activity.

Fixed doses of 120 or 240mg metoprolol daily were reported by Bengtsson (1976a) to be significantly more effective than placebo in reducing diastolic and systolic blood pressure in all positions in 23 women who had previously been treated with β-adrenoceptor blocking drugs. There was a tendency for blood pressure to be lower with a dose of 240mg metoprolol daily than with half this dose, but the difference was not significant. In the study reported by Waal-Manning (1976b), supine blood pressure was 162/97mm Hg after 3 weeks on placebo and 143/86 after 3 weeks' treatment with an individually determined dose of metoprolol. Corresponding values for standing blood pressure were 152/100 and 135/88mm Hg for placebo and metoprolol respectively. During mental arithmetic, sitting blood pressure was 182/115 with placebo and 171/108 with metoprolol. These differences between placebo and active therapy were statistically significant.

5.2 Comparison with Other Drugs

Metoprolol in fixed (Bosman et al., 1977; Bengtsson, 1976b; Stokkeland et al., 1975) or in individually titrated doses (Davidson et al., 1976) has been shown to have antihypertensive activity similar to that of other β-adrenoceptor blocking drugs at equivalent β-blocking dosages, and to α-methyldopa (Bergstrand et al., 1976) and hydrochlorothiazine (Pedersen, 1976), and superior to that of relatively low doses of trichlormethiazide (Stokkeland et al., 1975).

In a double-blind study (Davidson et al., 1976) in 25 patients with stable, uncomplicated, essential hypertension, individually titrated doses of metoprolol were compared with titrated doses of propranolol, oxprenolol, practolol and tolamolol (Davidson et al., 1976). At the end of an initial dose-finding period the average dosages and dose range of the drugs were propranolol 540mg (160 to 1280), oxprenolol 580mg (160 to 1280), practolol 720mg (400 to 1600), tolamolol 480mg (200 to 800) and metoprolol 380mg (100 to 800). All drugs were given twice daily.

Compared with values on placebo, all drugs produced a statistically significant and similar reduction in blood pressure. Reductions were greater for systolic than diastolic pressure and greatest during a high level of exercise (fig. 4). There were no significant differences between the blood pressure lowering activities of the various drugs with the exception of tolamolol which produced a greater reduction than the others in standing blood pressure. This may possibly result from its weak intrinsic vasodilator activity. Heart rate was reduced more by metoprolol and propranolol, drugs without intrinsic β-adrenoceptor agonist activity, than by the other drugs except during the higher level of exercise.

No statistically significant difference between the antihypertensive activity of metoprolol 50 or 100mg 3 times daily and 40 or 80mg propranolol 3 times daily was found by Bengtsson (1976b) in 23 women who had previously taken β-adrenoceptor blocking drugs. The same patients had been studied by Bengtsson in a previous placebo controlled investigation (1976a). The blood pressure was ≤ 140/90mm Hg in 9 on metoprolol and in 10 on propranolol.

A different result was reported by Bosman et al. (1977) in a multicentre between-patient comparison of propranol and metoprolol involving 81 patients from 4 centres in South Africa. These patients, with a resting diastolic blood pressure of 105 to 125mm Hg before treatment, were allocated at random to receive metoprolol 120mg, metoprolol 210mg, propranolol 240mg or propranolol 360mg daily. The treatment groups were not significantly different with regard to age, sex, body weight, duration of hypertension, diagnosis or previous antihypertensive medication. Metoprolol 120mg daily was superior to propranolol at either dose level in maintaining supine diastolic blood pressure at 90 to 95mm Hg or less. A trend in the same

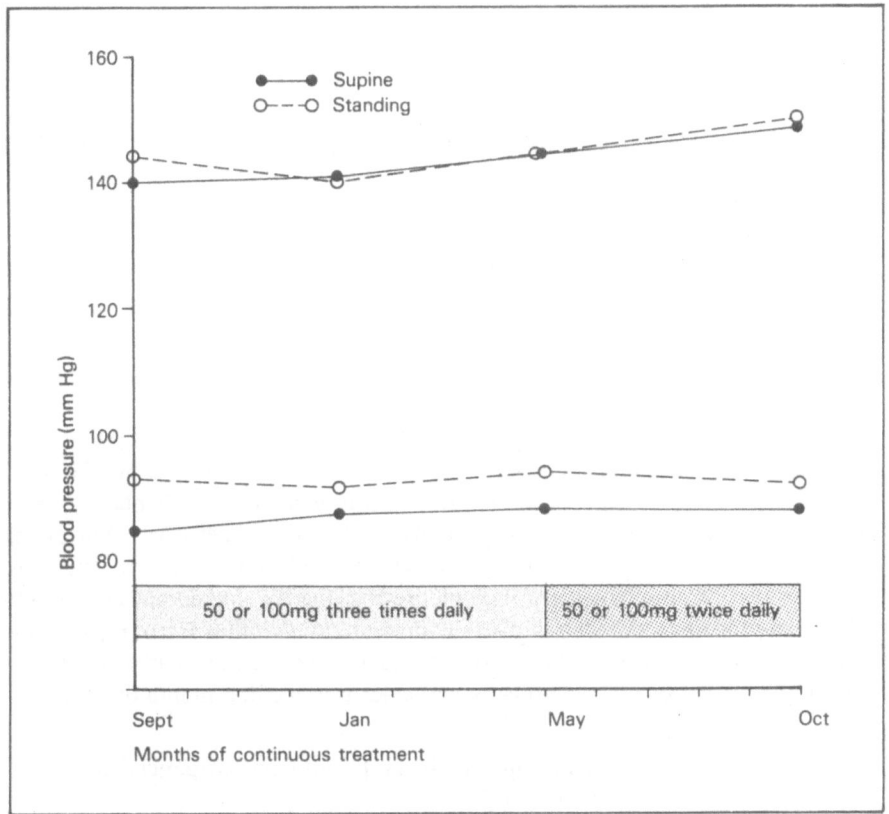

Fig. 4. Supine and standing systolic and diastolic blood pressure during thrice and twice daily regimens of metoprolol in 23 patients with moderate or mild essential hypertension (compiled from data in Bengtsson, 1976a).

direction was found for erect diastolic pressure, but this did not reach the level of statistical significance until the results with both dosages of metoprolol were pooled. Diastolic and systolic blood pressure was significantly reduced by 6 weeks of treatment with all regimens, except propranolol 360mg.

Bergstrand et al. (1976) reported that metoprolol in individually titrated doses of up to 450mg daily exerted a hypotensive effect comparable with that of α-methyldopa in doses of up to 2,250mg daily in 32 male patients with previously untreated essential hypertension.

In comparisons of metoprolol and thiazide diuretics, metoprolol 150 to 300mg daily has been shown to be comparable with hydrochlorothiazide 50 to 100mg daily (Pedersen, 1976) and superior to trichlormethiazide 2 to 4mg daily (Stokkeland et al., 1975). In the later study, however, the fixed dose of trichlormethiazide may have been too low to produce an effect on blood pressure comparable with that of metoprolol at the dosages chosen.

5.3 Metoprolol Combined with Other Drugs

Metoprolol 150 or 300mg daily alone or combined with hydrallazine 75 or 150mg daily was reported by Tuomilehto and Pakarinen (1977) to be effective in reducing sitting diastolic blood pressure to less than 95mm Hg (9) or by more than 10% (6) in 15 of 17 patients who had failed to respond to previous antihypertensive therapy. Nine patients responded satisfactorily to metoprolol alone whilst a further 6 patients achieved a satisfactory response with the combined regimen.

5.4 Long Term Treatment of Hypertension

Studies in which metoprolol alone in individually titrated doses of up to 450mg daily has been given for periods of 3 months or more (Hansson et al., 1977a,b; Rosengard, 1977) have reported a significant fall in blood pressure which has been maintained throughout the study. In a multicentre trial (Rosengard, 1977) involving 76 patients with previously untreated hypertension and 61 patients who were unsatisfactorily controlled by, or intolerant of, previous therapy, metoprolol alone (75 to 450mg daily) led to a decrease in diastolic pressure to $\leqslant$ 95mm Hg in 62% of the previously untreated group and in 50% of those previously treated with other drugs. Most of the reduction in blood pressure was evident in the first month of treatment.

5.5 Is the Efficacy of Metoprolol in Hypertension Influenced by Frequency of Administration?

Once daily metoprolol appears to be comparable in efficacy to a twice or thrice daily regimen in which the same total dose is given, in reducing blood pressure in patients with mild to moderate hypertension, although the thrice daily regimen tended to have a more potent and less fluctuating hypotensive action (Reybrouck et al., 1978).

In a well designed double-blind cross-over study in 16 hypertensive patients, Reybrouck et al. (1978) found that metoprolol 300mg given as a single daily dose lowered blood pressure to an extent not significantly different from that achieved with 100mg thrice daily. Plasma drug concentrations and the degree of β-blockade varied considerably throughout the day on the single dose regimen. These authors concluded that a once daily dosage of 300mg could be used if the only aim was to reduce blood pressure, but not if a steady degree of β-blockade was needed. A single daily dose of 300mg metoprolol alone produced a satisfactory reduction of blood pressure in 16 of 33 patients (Bloem et al., 1978). The addition of 37.5mg of hydrochlorothiazide reduced the blood pressure to < 94mm Hg in a further 8 patients.

In a comparison of metoprolol (200mg) and sotolol (240mg) Lehtonen and Sundquist (1978) found that both drugs had a similar and significant hypotensive effect when administered as a single daily dose. Sotolol effectively lowered blood pressure when given as a single dose on alternate days, but metoprolol had no effect on systolic blood pressure when given once in 48 hours.

Bengtsson (1976a) reduced the frequency of administration from thrice to twice daily in patients whose blood pressure had already been controlled with a thrice daily regimen. In this study the dosage as well as the frequency of administration was reduced (150 to 100mg and 300 to 200mg) but there was little difference in mean blood pressure after the change to the twice daily regimen (fig. 4). The frequency of administration was subsequently reduced to once daily (Bengtsson, 1976c), the dosage being unaltered. Over a 5-month period, blood pressure remained well controlled in 21 of the 24 patients. Two patients resumed the twice daily regimen because of side effects on once daily dosage, and one because of loss of blood pressure control. Further data (Johnsson, personal communication 1977; Gordon, 1976) suggest that in most patients studied, moderately elevated blood pressure can be satisfactorily controlled by once daily administration of metoprolol.

It has still to be shown in suitably designed studies in adequate numbers of patients, that *initial* treatment of elevated blood pressure with once or twice daily metoprolol results in reduction of blood pressure equal to that achieved with a thrice daily regimen. Such studies are required, particularly in severe hypertension.

Although Davidson et al., (1976) found that metoprolol and other β-adrenoceptor blocking drugs successfully controlled blood pressure when given twice daily, it may be that the blood pressure would have been lowered further if a thrice daily regimen were used. So far there are no published studies of the treatment of severe blood pressure with metoprolol, thus it cannot be determined if a thrice daily regimen is preferable to less frequent administration in such patients. In such cases, the frequency of administration of metoprolol will probably be governed to some extent by the timing of administration of concurrent medication to control blood pressure.

5.6 What is the Role of Metoprolol in Hypertension?

Studies with metoprolol indicate that it is as effective in lowering elevated blood pressure as any other β-adrenoceptor blocking drug given in a dose which produces a similar reduction in exercise-induced increase in heart rate (i.e. at equi-β-blocking doses). Metoprolol is as suitable as any other β-adrenoceptor blocking drug in the treatment of hypertension in patients in whom the use of these drugs is considered appropriate. Once daily dosage is effective in lowering blood pressure, but if a steady degree of β-blockade is desired a single daily dose of metoprolol cannot be recommended (Reybrouck et al., 1978).

As metoprolol is a β_1-selective adrenoceptor blocking drug (sections 3.3.1 and 3.3.2), along with other 'cardioselective' drugs of this class it may cause less tendency to impair peripheral circulation, heart failure and hypertensive reactions in states of catecholamine excess. 'Cardioselectivity' lessens the risk of bronchospasm, but does not impart any advantage with regard to its antihypertensive action. Metoprolol may be better than non-selective β-adrenoceptor blocking drugs in the treatment of hypertension in patients who also experience Raynaud's phenomenon. β_1-Adrenoceptor selectivity may possibly also be an advantage in patients with diabetes mellitus, who are receiving insulin or oral hypoglycaemic agents (section 3.5.1), and those with angina or heart failure controlled by diuretics and digitalis drugs, but conclusive evidence for any advantage of β_1-selective agents in these conditions has yet to be demonstrated. Metoprolol is not suitable in patients who are in need of a β_1-selective drug with partial agonist activity (e.g. patients at risk from A-V conduction impairment), but its lack of partial agonist activity may be of value in patients with muscle cramps (Waal-Manning, 1976c), thyrotoxicosis (Turner, 1974), or in those who have a high-dose hypertensive response to pindolol (Waal-Manning, 1976c). As with other β-adrenoceptor blocking drugs, metoprolol is probably best given along with a diuretic and vasodilator in the more severe cases of hypertension (Waal-Manning, 1976c).

Metoprolol has somewhat less effect on basal FEV_1 in asthmatic patients than equiactive doses of propranolol, but still has a clinically significant effect at doses of 200mg daily. Thus, like other β-adrenoceptor blocking drugs metoprolol, at doses usually necessary to control elevated blood pressure, is best avoided in patients with asthma. Since metoprolol is selective in its effect on β-adrenoceptors and does not inhibit the action of β_2-adrenoceptor stimulating drugs on the airways, where it is considered absolutely necessary, small doses of metoprolol (up to 100mg daily) can be used with extreme caution in patients with asthma or bronchitis and bronchospasm.

Such patients must also receive optimum regular treatment with a β_2-adrenoceptor stimulant drug such as terbutaline, salbutamol, etc. (see also section 8).

6. Side Effects

In therapeutic trials in patients with hypertension, metoprolol has been well tolerated and any side effects reported have been moderate or mild and have generally not interfered with normal daily activities.

In studies that have employed questionnaires with lists of possible side effects, the frequency of adverse effects has been similar during placebo and metoprolol (Ekelund et al., 1976; Frick and Luurila, 1976; Keyrilainen and Uusitalo 1975, 1976).

During a 6-month study in patients with angina pectoris (Keyrilainen and Uusilato, 1976), a greater proportion of side effects (33%) interfered with normal daily activity during the first month than at 3 months (18%) and 6 months (17%). In this study, tiredness, insomnia, and gastric upset were the most frequently reported side effects with metoprolol during long term treatment, although during subsequent double-blind comparison with placebo in the same patients, the frequency of these and other side effects on the check list were similar during both periods. Nevertheless, dizziness and tiredness have been the most frequently reported side effects in some other studies (Jaattela and Pyorala, 1976; Bengtsson 1976a).

Venous congestion parallel to an increase in heart volume was reported in 1 patient by Frick and Luurila (1976). There have been no reports of cardiac failure, but in some studies patients at risk have been excluded. The oculo-mucocutaneous and various autoimmune reactions seen with practolol have not been reported with metoprolol, but relatively few patients have been studied for 23 months, the mean time for induction of the eye signs in the practolol cases (Dollery, 1976). Peyronie's disease possibly associated with metoprolol has been reported in 1 patient (Yudkin, 1977) as has peripheral gangrene (Vale and Jefferys, 1978).

7. Contraindications

Metoprolol should not be used if there is a risk of congestive heart failure, unless the patient is satisfactorily controlled with a diuretic and/or digitalis, and then given only cautiously; nor should it be used in patients with right ventricular failure secondary to pulmonary hypertension. Significant cardiomegaly of any cause is an indication for considerable caution, as with other β-adrenoceptor blocking drugs.

The drug should not be used in patients with sinus bradycardia (rate of less than 60 per minute) unless the patient is being paced, in patients with second or third degree atrioventricular block, or in patients with cardiogenic shock.

If anaesthesia is required in patients taking metoprolol, the anaesthetic should be one that does not cause myocardial depression.

8. Precautions

As with other β-adrenoceptor blocking drugs, patients with mild or latent cardiac insufficiency should be given a diuretic and/or adequate doses of digitalis prior to receiving metoprolol.

Metoprolol may be administered with caution to patients with bronchitis and a tendency to wheezing, provided that bronchodilator therapy with a β_2-adrenoceptor stimulant drug such as terbutaline, salbutamol etc. is administered concomitantly. Although it is best to avoid any β-adrenoceptor blocking drug in asthma, some consider that low doses of metoprolol (up to 100mg daily) may be given if it is thought essential in asthmatic patients, who must also be receiving optimum regular therapy with β_2-adrenoceptor stimulants. It may be necessary to increase the dose of β_2-stimulant or institute combined oral and inhalation therapy in these patients.

Metoprolol therapy must be reported to the anaesthetist prior to general anaesthesia for surgery.

Caution should be observed when treating patients with unstable diabetes mellitus, as adjustment of the dose of the hypoglycaemic agent may be necessary.

Pending further clinical experience, metoprolol is not recommended for use during pregnancy.

9. Dosage

Initially, 25 to 50mg night and morning. This dose may be increased to 100 to 200mg twice daily depending on the response. Higher doses of up to about 400mg daily may be given if required. The dosage required to control blood pressure can be given once daily in many patients with mild to moderate hypertension. Metoprolol may be given as part of a combined treatment regimen with a diuretic and/or a third drug (such as a peripheral vasodilator) where combined therapy is necessary to control blood pressure.

10. Overdosage

A case of massive intoxication with metoprolol has been reported (Moeller, 1976) in a 19-year-old male who ingested 10,000mg (160mg/kg). The plasma level was 12,200ng/g plasma at 2 hours after hospital admission and 9,400ng/g and 5,700ng/g at 7 and 10 hours respectively. Initial treatment was gastric lavage, infusion of balanced electrolyte solution and sodium bicarbonate and control of blood pressure (which was not registrable) with metaraminol. After these measures, the patient was comfortable and without signs of cardiovascular depression 12 hours after admission.

Acknowledgements

Various sections of the manuscript reviewed by: *C. Bengtsson*, Medical Department, University of Goteborg, Sweden; *J.S. Borer*, National Heart, Lung and Blood Institute, Bethesda, Maryland, USA; *J.P. Chalmers*, Flinders Medical Centre, Bedford Park, Australia; *C. Davidson*, Birch Hill Hospital, Rochdale, England; *L.-C. Ekelund*, Karolinska Institutet, Stockholm, Sweden; *A.S.P. Hua*, Department of Medicine, Royal Melbourne Hospital, Victoria, Australia; *A. Jaattela*, Department of Medicine, University of Helsinki, Helsinki, Finland; *R.J. Newman*, Department of Anatomy, University of Leeds, Leeds, England; *F.O. Simpson*, University of Otago, Dunedin, New Zealand; *G.S. Stokes*, Cardio-Renal Unit, Sydney Hospital, Sydney, Australia; *G. Thiringer*, Renstromska Sjukhuset, Goteborg, Sweden; *H.J. Waal-Manning*, Wellcome Medical Research Institute, University of Otago, Dunedin; *R. Zacest*, Department of Clinical Pharmacology, Queen Elizabeth Hospital, Woodville, Australia.

References

Ablad, B.; Carlsson, B.; Carlsson, E.; Dahlof, C.; Ek, L. and Hultberg, E.: Cardiac effects of β-adrenergic receptor antagonists. Advances in Cardiology 12: 290 (1974).

Ablad, B.; Carlsson, E and Ek, L.: Pharmacological studies of two new cardioselective adrenergic beta-receptor antagonists. Life Sciences 12: 107 (1973).

Appelgren, C.; Borg, K.O.; Elofsson, R. and Johansson, K.A.: Binding of adrenergic beta-receptor antagonists to human serum albumin. Acta Pharmaceutica Suecica 11: 329 (1974).

Arfwidsson, A.; Borg, K.O.; Hoffmann, K-J. and Skanberg, I.: Metabolism of metoprolol in the rat *in vitro* and *in vivo*. Xenobiotica 6: 691 (1976).

Attman, P.O.; Aurell, M. and Johnsson, G.: Effects of metoprolol and propranolol and furosemide-stimulated renin release in healthy subjects. European Journal of Clinical Pharmacology 8: 201 (1975).

Bahr, C. von.; Collste, P.; Frisk-Holmberg, M; Haglund, K.; Jorfelt, L.; Orme, M.; Ostman, J. and Sjoqvist, F.: Plasma levels and effects of metoprolol on blood pressure, adrenergic beta receptor blockade and plasma renin activity in essential hypertension. Clinical Pharmacology and Therapeutics 20: 130 (1976).

Bengtsson, C.: The effect of metoprolol — a new selective adrenergic β_1-receptor blocking agent — in mild hypertension. Acta Medica Scandinavica 199: 65 (1976a).

Bengtsson, C.: Comparison between metoprolol and propranolol as antihypertensive agents. Acta Medica Scandinavica 199: 71 (1976b).

Bengtsson, C.: Treatment with beta-blockers — significance of dose and number of administrations. Translation of abstract from 35th Scandinavian Congress of Internal Medicine 9-11th June 1976, Finland (1976c).

Bengtsson, C.; Johnsson, G. and Regardh, C.-G.: Plasma levels and effects of metoprolol on blood
    pressure and heart rate in hypertensive patients after an acute dose and between two doses during
    long-term treatment. Clinical Pharmacology and Therapeutics 17: 400 (1975).
Bergstrand, R.H.; Vedin, J.A.; Wilhelmsson, C.E. and Berglund, G.: Comparative study of metoprolol
    and alpha-methyldopa in untreated essential hypertension. European Journal of Clinical Pharma-
    cology 10: 375 (1976).
Benson, M.K.; Berrill, W.T.; Sterling, G.M.; Decalmer, P.B.; Chatterjee, S.S.; Croxson, R.S. and
    Cruickshank, J.M.: Cardioselective and non-cardioselective beta-blockers in reversible obstructive
    airways disease. Postgraduate Medical Journal 53 (Suppl. 3): 143 (1977).
Bloem, Th. J.J.M.; Disch, R.P.; Lindren, P.C.J.M. and Kerkhof, J.V.D.: Anithypertensive effects of
    metoprolol and a fixed-ratio combination of metoprolol and hydrochlorothiazide given once daily.
    Current Therapeutic Research 24: 26 (1978).
Bodin, N.-O; Borg, K.O.; Johansson, R.; Ramsay, C.H. and Skanberg, I.: Tissue distribution of
    metoprolol-(3H) in the mouse and the rat. Acta Pharmacologica et Toxicologica 36 (Suppl. V): 116
    (1975a).
Bodin, N.-O; Flodh, H.; Magnusson, G.; Malmfors, T. and Nyberg, J-A: Toxicological studies on
    metoprolol. Acta Pharmacologica et Toxicologica 36 (Suppl. V): 96 (1975b).
Borg, K.O.; Carlsson, E.; Ek, L. and Johansson, R.: Combined pharmacokinetic and pharmacodynamic
    studies of metoprolol in the cat and the dog. Acta Pharmacologica et Toxicologica 36 (Suppl. V): 24
    (1975a).
Borg, K.O.; Carlsson, E.; Hoffmann, K-J; Jansson, T-E; Thorin, H. and Wallin, B.: Metabolism of
    metoprolol-(3H) in man, the dog and the rat. Acta Pharmacologica et Toxicologica 36
    (Suppl. V): 125 (1975c).
Borg, K.O.; Fellenius, E.; Johansson, R. and Wallborg, M.: Pharmacokinetic studies of metoprolol-(^{3}H) in
    the rat and the dog. Acta Pharmacologica et Toxicologica 36 (Suppl. V): 104 (1975b).
Bosman, A.R.; Goldberg, B.; McKechnies, J.K.; Offermeier, J. and Oosthuizen, O.J.: South African Mul-
    ticentre study of metoprolol and propranolol in essential hypertension. South African Medical Jour-
    nal 51: 57 (1977).
Comerford, M.B. and Besterman, E.M.M.: Relative activity of atenolol and metoprolol. British Medical
    Journal 2: 260 (1977).
Davidson, C.; Thadani, U.; Singleton, W. and Taylor, S.H.: Comparison of antihypertensive activity of
    beta-blocking drugs during chronic treatment. British Medical Journal 2: 7 (1976).
Davidson, N. McD.; Corrall, R.J.M.; Shaw, T.R.D. and French, E.B.: Observations in man of hypo-
    glycaemia during selective and non-selective beta-blockade. Scottish Medical Journal 22: 69 (1977).
Davies, C.P.; Kendall, M.J. and John, V.A.: Comparison of plasma and saliva levels of metoprolol and
    oxprenolol. British Journal of Clinical Pharmacology 5: 217 (1978).
Dollery, C.T.: Closing remarks. Current status of labetalol. British Journal of Clinical Pharmacology 3
    (Suppl.): 823 (1976).
Ekberg, G. and Hansson, B-G.: Glucose tolerance and insulin release in hypertensive patients treated with
    the cardioselective β-receptor blocking agent metoprolol. Acta Medica Scandinavica 202: 393
    (1977).
Ekelund, L.-G.; Olsson, A.G.; Oro, L. and Rossner, S.: Effects of the cardioselective beta-adrenergic
    receptor blocking agent metoprolol in angina pectoris. Subacute study with exercise tests. British
    Heart Journal 38: 155 (1976).
Formgren, H.: The effect of metoprolol and practolol on lung function and blood pressure in hypertensive
    asthmatics. British Journal of Clinical Pharmacology 3: 1007 (1976).
Frick, M.H. and Luurila, O.: Double-blind titrated dose comparison of metoprolol and propranolol in the
    treatment of angina pectoris. Annals of Clinical Research 8: 385 (1976).
Gordon, R.D.: Initial treatment of the young hypertensive: thiazide diuretic or β-adrenoreceptor-blocking
    agent in a single daily dose? Clinical Science and Molecular Medicine 51: 631s-633s (1976).

Hansson, B.-G.; Dymling, J.-F.; Hedeland, H. and Hulthen, U.L.: Long-term treatment of moderate hypertension with the beta₁-receptor blocking agent metoprolol. 1. Effect of maximal working capacity, plasma catecholamines and renin, urinary aldosterone, blood pressure and pulse rate under basal conditions. European Journal of Clinical Pharmacology 11: 239 (1977a).

Hansson, B.-G.; Dymling, J.-F.; Manhem, P. and Hokfelt, B.: Long-term treatment of moderate hypertension with the beta₁-receptor blocking agent metoprolol. II. Effect of submaximal work and insulin-induced hypoglycaemia on plasma catecholamines and renin activity, blood pressure and pulse rate. European Journal of Clinical Pharmacology 11: 247 (1977b).

Harms, H.H.; Gooren, L.; Spoelstra, A.J.G.; Hesse, C. and Versehoor, L.: Blockade of isoprenaline-induced changes in plasma free fatty acids, immunoreactive insulin levels and plasma renin activity in healthy human subjects, by propranolol, pindolol, practolol, atenolol, metoprolol and acebutolol. British Journal of Clinical Pharmacology 5: 19 (1978).

van Herwaarden, C.L.A.; Binkhorst, R.A.; Fennis, J.F.M. and van't Laar, A.: Effects of adrenaline during treatment with propranolol and metoprolol. British Medical Journal 1: 1029 (1977).

van Herwaarden, C.L.A.; Ferris, J.F.M.; Binkhorst, R.A. and van't Laar, A.: Haemodynamic effects of adrenaline during treatment of hypertensive patients with propranolol and metoprolol. European Journal of Clinical Pharmacology 12: 397 (1977).

Hokfelt, B.; Hansson, B-G.; Heding, L.G. and Nilsson, K.O.: Effect of insulin induced hypoglycaemia on the blood levels of catecholamines, glucagon, growth hormone, cortisol, C-peptide and proinsulin before and during medication with the cardioselective beta-receptor blocking agent metoprolol in man. Acta Endocrinologica 87: 659 (1978).

Horvath, J.; Woolcock, A.; Tiller, D. and Caterson, R.: The effects of metoprolol and propranolol on hypertension and respiratory function in patients with hypertension and normal lung function. Australian and New Zealand Journal of Medicine 7: 445 (1977).

Hunyor, S. and Nyberg, G.: Comparison of intra-arterial and indirect blood pressures at rest and during isometric exercise in hypertensive patients before and after metoprolol. British Journal of Clinical Pharmacology 6: 109 (1978).

Jaattela, A. and Pyorala, K.: A controlled study on the antihypertensive effect of a new β-adrenergic receptor blocking drug, metoprolol, in combination with chlorthalidone. British Journal of Clinical Pharmacology 3: 655 (1976).

Johansson, K.A.; Appelgren, C.; Borg, K.O. and Elofsson, R.: Binding of two adrenergic beta-receptor antagonists, alprenolol and H93/26, to human serum proteins. Acta Pharm. Suec. 11: 333 (1974).

Johnsson, G.: Influence of metoprolol and propranolol on haemodynamic effects induced by adrenaline and physical work. Acta Pharmacologica et Toxicologica 36 (Suppl. V): 59 (1975a).

Johnsson, G.: Selectivity studies with adrenergic β-receptor blockers in man, in Pathophysiology and Management of Arterial Hypertension, Proceedings of a Conference Copenhagen, Denmark, April 10-11 (1975b).

Johnsson (personal communication) Clinical documentation for a once daily regimen of metoprolol in the treatment of hypertension (unpublished data).

Johnsson, G. and Regardh, C.-G.: Clinical pharmacokinetics of β-adrenoreceptor blocking drugs. Clinical Pharmacokinetics 1: 233 (1976).

Johnsson, G.; Nyberg, G. and Solvell, L.: Influence of metoprolol and propranolol on hemodynamic effects induced by physical work and isoprenaline. Acta Pharmacologica et Toxicologica 36 (Suppl. V): 69 (1975b).

Johnsson, G.; Regardh, C.-G. and Solvell, L.: Combined pharmacokinetic and pharmacodynamic studies in man of the adrenergic β₁-receptor antagonist metoprolol. Acta Pharmacologica et Toxicologica 36 (Suppl. V): 31 (1975a).

Johnsson, G.; Svedmyr, N. and Thiringer, G.: Effects of intravenous propranolol and metoprolol and their interaction with isoprenaline on pulmonary function, heart rate and blood pressure in asthmatics. European Journal of Clinical Pharmacology 8: 175 (1975c).

Keyrilainen, O. and Uusitalo, A.: Effects of the cardioselective beta-blocker metoprolol in angina pectoris. Annals of Clinical Research 7: 433 (1975).

Keyrilainen, O. and Uusitalo, A.: Effects of metoprolol in angina pectoris. Acta Medica Scandinavica 199: 491 (1976).

Lehtonen, A. and Sundquist, H.: Comparison of antihypertensive activity of sotolol and metoprolol administered once daily and every other day. Current Therapeutic Research 23: 131 (1978).

Ljung, B.; Ablad, B.; Drews, L.; Fellenius, E.: Kjellstedt, A. and Wallborg, M.: Antihypertensive effect of metoprolol in spontaneously hypertensive rats. Clinical Science and Molecular Medicine 51: 443 (1976).

Loubatieres, A.; Mariani, M.M.; Sorel, G. and Savi, L.: The action of β-adrenergic blocking and stimulating agents on insulin secretion. Characterisation of the type of β-receptor. Diabetologica 7: 127 (1971).

Lundborg, P. and Steen, B.: Plasma levels and effect on heart rate and blood pressure of metoprolol, after acute oral administration in 12 geriatric patients. Acta Medica Scandinavica 5: 397 (1976).

Lundgren, B.: Comparison of two β_1-selective blockers, atenolol and metoprolol, in the reserpinised cat. Acta Pharmacologica et Toxicologica 41 (Suppl. 4): 62 (1977).

Lund-Johansen, P. and Ohm, O.J.: Haemodynamic long-term effects of β-receptor blocking agents in hypertension: a comparison between alprenolol, atenolol, metoprolol and timolol. Clinical Science and Molecular Medicine 51: 481S (1976).

Lund-Johansen, P. and Ohm, O.J.: Haemodynamic long-term effects of metoprolol at rest and during exercise in essential hypertension. British Journal of Clinical Pharmacology 3: 147 (1977).

Moeller, B.H.: Massive intoxication with metoprolol. British Medical Journal 1: 222 (1976).

Newman, R.J.: Comparison of propranolol, metoprolol and acebutolol on insulin-induced hypoglycaemia. British Medical Journal 2: 447 (1976).

Nilsson, A.; Hansson, B.-G. and Hokfelt, B.: Effect of beta$_1$-receptor blockade (metoprolol) on the blood content of catecholamines, glycerol, free fatty acids, triglycerides and glucose in hypertensive patients during rest and following submaximal work. European Journal of Clinical Pharmacology 13: 5 (1978).

Nyberg, G.: Effect of β-adrenoreceptor blockers on heart rate and blood pressure in dynamic and isometric exercises. Drugs 11 (Suppl. 1): 185 (1976).

Pedersen, O.L.: Comparison of metoprolol and hydrochlorothiazide as antihypertensive agents. European Journal of Clinical Pharmacology 10: 381 (1976).

Pfisterer, M.; Burkart, F.; Buhler, F.R. and Schweizer, W.: Hamodynamische veranderungen unter metoprolol bei hypertension patienten in vergleich zu propranolol. Schweizerische Medizinische Wochenschrift 106: 1567 (1976).

Prichard, B.N.C.: β-Adrenergic receptor blocking drugs in angina pectoris. Drugs 7: 55 (1974).

Regardh, C.-G; Borg, K.O.; Johansson, R.; Johnsson, G. and Palmer, L.: Pharmacokinetic studies on the selective β_1 receptor antagonist metoprolol in man. Journal of Pharmacokinetics and Biopharmaceutics 2: 347 (1974).

Regardh, C.-G; Johnsson, G.; Jordo, L. and Solvell, L.: Comparative bioavailability and effect studies on metoprolol administered as ordinary and slow-release tablets in single and multiple doses. Acta Pharmacologica et Toxicologica 36 (Suppl. V): 45 (1975).

Reybrouck, T.; Amery, A.; Fagard, R.; Jousten, P.; Lijnen, P. and Meulepas, E.: Beta-Blockers: once or three times a day. British Medical Journal 1: 1386 (1978).

Rosengard, S.: Antihypertensive effect and tolerability for metoprolol during long-term treatment: A multicentre study. Journal of International Medical Research 5: 199 (1977).

Ruskoaho, H. and Karppanen, H.: Inhibition of the development of spontaneous hypertension in rats by metoprolol. Acta Pharmacologica et Toxicologica 41 (Suppl. 4): 72 (1977).

Sannerstedt, R. and Wasir, H.: Acute haemodynamic effects of metoprolol in hypertensive patients. British Journal of Clinical Pharmacology 4: 23 (1977).

Singh, B.N.; Whitlock, R.M.L.; Comber, R.H.; Williams, F.H. and Harris, E.A.: Effects of cardioselective beta adrenoceptor blockade on specific airways resistance in normal subjects and in patients with bronchial asthma. Clinical Pharmacology and Therapeutics 19: 493 (1976).

Skinner, C.; Gaddie, J.; Palmer, K.N.V. and Kerridge, D.F.: Comparison of effect of metoprolol and propranolol on asthmatic airway obstruction. British Medical Journal 1: 504 (1976).

Stenberg, J.; Wasir, H.; Amery, A.; Sannerstedt, R. and Werko, L.: Comparative hemodynamic studies in man of adrenergic β_1-receptor agents without (H93/26 = metoprolol) or with (H87/07) intrinsic sympathicomimetic activity. Acta Pharmacologica et Toxicologica 36 (Suppl. V): 76 (1975).

Stokkeland, O.M.; Sangvik, K. and Lindseth Ditlefsen, E.-M.: A comparative study of metoprolol and trichlormethiazide in hypertension. Current Therapeutic Research 18: 755 (1975).

Thiringer, G. and Svedmyr, N.: Interaction of orally administered metoprolol, practolol, and propranolol with isoprenaline in asthmatics. European Journal of Clinical Pharmacology 10: 163 (1976).

Tivenius, L.: Effects of multiple doses of metoprolol and propranolol on ventilatory function in patients with chronic obstructive lung disease. Scandinavian Journal of Respiratory Diseases 57: 190 (1976).

Tuomilehto, J. and Pakarinen, P.: Effects of metoprolol as monotherapy and in combination with hydrallazine in hypertensive patients previously considered to be treatment failures. Current Therapeutic Research 21: 257 (1977).

Turner, P.: β-Adrenergic receptor blocking drugs in hyperthyroidism. Drugs 7: 48 (1974).

Vale, J.A. and Jefferys, D.B.: Peripheral gangrene complicating beta-blockade. Lancet 1: 1216 (1978).

Waal-Manning, H.J.: Metabolic effects of β-adrenoreceptor blockers. Drugs 11 (Suppl. 1): 121 (1976a).

Waal-Manning, H.J.: Experience with β-adrenoreceptor blockers in hypertension. Drugs 11 (Suppl. 1): 164 (1976b).

Waal-Manning, H.J.: Hypertension: Which β-blocker. Drugs 12: 412 (1976c).

Weiss, L.; Lundgren, Y. and Folkow, B.: Effects of prolonged treatment with adrenergic β-receptor antagonists on blood pressure, cardiovascular design and reactivity in spontaneously hypertensive rats (SHR). Acta Physiologica Scandinavica 91: 447 (1974).

Wood, A.J.: Cerebrospinal fluid concentration of metoprolol in a hypertensive patient. British Journal of Clinical Pharmacology 4: 240 (1977).

Yudkin, J.S.: Peyronie's disease in association with metoprolol. Lancet 2: 1355 (1977).

Chapter III

Labetalol: A Review of its Pharmacology and Therapeutic Use in Hypertension

R.N. Brogden, R.C. Heel, T.M. Speight and G.S. Avery

1. Pharmacology

Labetalol is a salicylamide derivative (fig. 1) synthesised by Dr L.H.C. Lunts and his colleagues which has been shown to be a specific competitive antagonist at both α- and β-adrenoceptors.

1.1 Blockade at α- and β-Adrenoceptors

In vitro and in isolated animal tissues (Aggerbeck et al., 1978; Blakeley and Summers, 1977; Farmer et al., 1972) and in intact animals (Farmer et al., 1972; Kennedy and Levy, 1975) labetalol is a competitive antagonist at α-adrenoceptors and is a non-selective antagonist at β-adrenoceptors (Harichaux and Hary, 1976). Labetalol has no intrinsic agonist (sympathomimetic) activity at β-adrenoceptors (Farmer et al., 1972). At doses higher than required for adrenoceptor blockade labetalol has some direct myocardial depressant action (Brittain and Levy, 1976), but this effect is not likely to be of clinical significance at the dosages used in the treatment of hypertension. Thus, at β_1-adrenoceptors, the characteristics of labetalol are most closely akin to those of propranolol, although it is less potent than propranolol (Farmer et al., 1972). In cat spleen, labetalol is an antagonist of postsynaptic α-adrenoceptors (Blakeley and Summers, 1976) and may thus resemble prazosin in its action at α-adrenoceptors (Cambridge et al., 1977). In isolated tissue studies, labetalol is 4 to 8 times more potent at β- than at α-adrenoceptors, whilst in anaesthetised dogs it is about 16 times more potent at cardiac β_1- than at vascular α-adrenoceptors (Farmer et al., 1972).

In man, labetalol given orally in single (Richards et al., 1976a,c) or multiple doses (Mehta and Cohn, 1977) or by intravenous injection (Collier et al., 1972; Richards et al., 1977b) has been shown to inhibit the effects of an infusion of isoprenaline (β-blockade) and of phenylephrine and noradrenaline (α-blockade) [Richards and Prichard, 1978]. As in animals, labetalol is more potent at β- than at α-receptors, the ratio being 3:1 after oral administration (Richards et al., 1976a,c) and 6.9:1 after intravenous labetalol (Richards et al., 1977b). In studies in superficial hand veins (Collier et al., 1972) the effect of labetalol in inhibiting noradrenaline in-duced constriction and the vasodilator response to isoprenaline was of short duration, and in direct contrast to the longer duration of effect after systemic administration of the drug (Collier et al., 1972). Oral labetalol 400mg significantly inhibited the venoconstrictor effect of locally infused phenylephrine into the veins of the hand (Richards, 1977). Propranolol was about 10 times more potent than labetalol in in-hibiting the venodilator response to locally infused isoprenaline (Collier et al., 1972), whilst after systemic administration the isoprenaline ratio was 3.8 after labetalol 10mg, 6.0 after 40mg and 37.4 after 160mg, and 13.2 after propranolol 10mg (Richards et al., 1977b). The differing magnitude of effects of propranolol and labetalol on heart rate, peak expiratory flow rate and diastolic blood pressure at rest (Richards et al., 1977a) were probably related to the additional α-adrenoceptor block-ing property of labetalol.

1.2 Haemodynamic Effects

In animals, observations of haemodynamic effects vary according to the experi-mental situation depending on the balance of autonomic influences (Brittain and

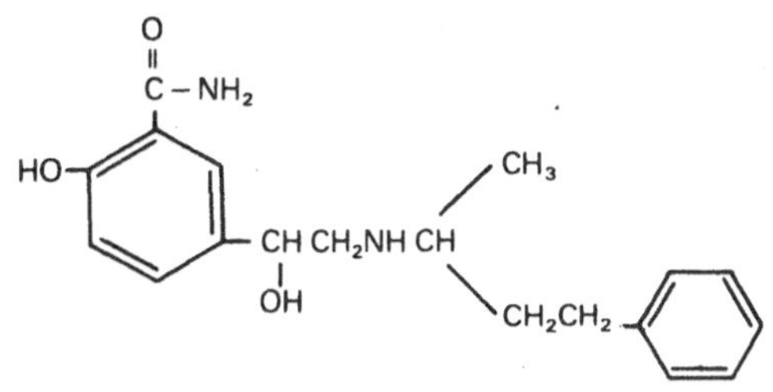

Fig. 1. Structural formula of labetalol.

Levy, 1976). Labetalol decreased heart rate and cardiac contractility, output and work
in some studies (Farmer et al., 1972) in anaesthetised dogs, but not in others (Maxwell, 1973). Unlike propranolol, acute administration of labetalol decreased total
peripheral vascular resistance. Compared with propranolol, labetalol caused larger
reductions in arterial blood pressure when given at equivalent β-blocking doses
(Farmer et al., 1972). In contrast to conventional β-blocking drugs, acute administration of labetalol reduces blood pressure in hypertensive animals (Brittain and Levy,
1976).

In man, acutely administered intravenous labetalol 50mg (Koch, 1976a, 1977)
or 0.5 to 1mg/kg (Joekes and Thompson, 1976; Prichard et al., 1975) reduced blood
pressure and peripheral vascular resistance and generally did not lower cardiac output
or stroke volume in the supine position (table I). Heart rate is not significantly altered
in supine resting hypertensive patients, but is significantly decreased in standing
patients and during exercise (Koch, 1976a, 1977). In hypertensive patients given
labetalol 300 to 1,200mg for a few days and up to 16 months, there is a significant
reduction in heart rate as well as in blood pressure (Andersson et al., 1976; Edwards
and Raftery, 1976; Koch, 1976b). The overall pattern of haemodynamic effects with
intravenous labetalol is similar to that observed (Prichard et al., 1975) after intravenous administration of a combination of propranolol (8 to 16mg) and hydrallazine

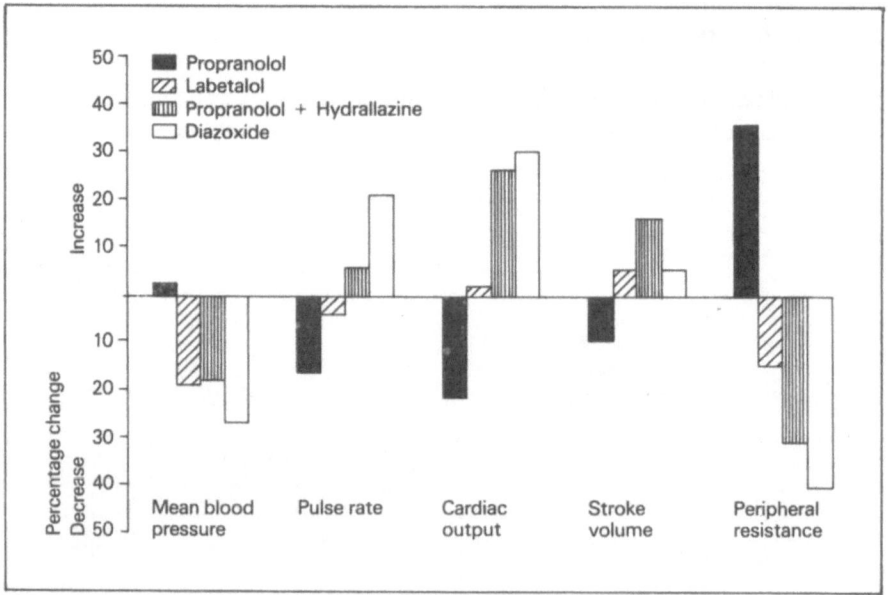

Fig. 2. Mean changes in haemodynamic variables in 12 hypertensive patients in response to
intravenous propranolol, labetalol, propranolol plus hydrallazine, and diazoxide (after Prichard et al.,
1975).

Table I. Effect of intravenous and oral labetalol on haemodynamic variables in hypertensive subjects

Author	No. pats	Dose labetalol	Effect[1]	BP[2]	HR	CO	PVR	SV
Intravenous administration								
Joekes and Thompson (1976)	14	50-100mg		↓	≒	≒	↓	≒
Koch (1976a, 1977)	13	50mg	Supine	↓	≒	≒	≒	...
			Upright	↓	↓	↓	↓	...
			Exercise	↓			↓	...
Prichard et al. (1975)	12	0.5mg/kg		↓	≒	≒	↓	≒
Oral administration								
Edwards and Raftery (1976)	11	800mg/d 4 weeks	Rest	↓	↓	≒	≒	↑
			Exercise (light)	↓	↓	≒	≒	↑
			Exercise (heavy)	↓	↓	↓	≒	≒
Mehta and Cohn (1977)	6	200 to 1,600mg daily. Dose doubled on successive days	Supine	↓	↓	≒	↓	...
			Upright	↓	↓	≒	↓	...

1   Effect relative to pretreatment values; ↓ = significant reduction; ↑ = significant increase, ≒ = no significant change.

2   Abbreviations: BP = blood pressure; HR = heart rate; CO = cardiac output; PVR = peripheral vascular resistance; SV = stroke volume.

(20mg), although labetalol has a less marked effect on cardiac output and peripheral resistance than that combination (fig. 2).

1.2.1 Effect on Blood Pressure and Heart Rate

A significant fall in systolic and diastolic blood pressure within 5 minutes of intravenous injection of labetalol 1 to 2mg/kg in resting hypertensive patients was reported by Rosei et al. (1976a), Trust et al. (1976) and Rønne-Rasmussen et al. (1976). A more rapid onset of hypotensive effect which was apparent in 1 minute and maximal at 3 minutes was reported in normal subjects given labetalol 1.5mg/kg intravenously (Richards et al., 1977b) and in patients given 2mg/kg by the same route

(Pearson and Havard, 1976). A maximum hypotensive response 20 to 40 minutes after a 0.5 to 1mg/kg dose given by infusion was noted by Joekes and Thompson (1976) in resting hypertensive patients. In hypertensive patients whose blood pressure was inadequately controlled by β-adrenoceptor blocking drugs, a significant fall in blood pressure was produced by labetalol 2mg/kg, but not by a dose of 1mg/kg. This finding may indicate that after intravenous injection the α-adrenoceptor blocking effect is predominant. After oral administration of single doses to normal subjects (Richards et al., 1974) blood pressure is significantly reduced, with the most marked falls occurring with higher doses. A hypotensive effect was apparent within 2 hours of oral labetalol in hypertensive subjects studied by Breckenridge et al. (1977a).

In studies comparing acutely administered labetalol with propranolol at one-fifth to one-half the dosage (Maconochie et al., 1977a,b; Prichard et al., 1975; Richards et al., 1977a) there has been a consistent significant fall in blood pressure with labetalol but not with propranolol. In a study (Prichard et al., 1975) comparing intravenous labetalol 0.5mg/kg with propranolol 8 to 16mg, with the same dose of propranolol plus 20mg hydrallazine, and with diazoxide 300mg, the pattern of haemodynamic effects was most akin to that of the combination of propranolol and hydrallazine (fig. 2), although changes in cardiac output and peripheral resistance were less marked with labetalol than with the combination.

Generally, changes in heart rate in resting supine patients or volunteers given intravenous labetalol have not been statistically significant, but in most studies in which labetalol has been given orally over a period of several days or longer there has been a significant reduction in heart rate (Andersson et al., 1976; Breckenridge et al., 1977a; Edwards and Raftery, 1976; Koch, 1976b; Mehta and Cohn, 1977; Richards et al., 1974). After intravenous or oral labetalol the decrease in heart rate has tended to be more pronounced in the upright position (Koch, 1976a, 1977; Mehta and Cohn, 1977) and during exercise (Richards et al., 1977b). Thus labetalol, at oral dosages likely to be used in the treatment of hypertension, can be expected to cause a decrease in heart rate of about 13 to 18% compared with baseline values.

1.2.2 Effect on Cardiac Output

In resting subjects with hypertension, oral (Edwards and Raftery, 1976; Mehta and Cohn, 1977) or intravenous labetalol (Joekes and Thompson, 1976; Koch, 1976a, 1977; Prichard et al., 1975) usually does not lower cardiac output although a significant reduction (18.2%) in the upright position following intravenous administration of labetalol 50mg in 13 hypertensive patients was reported by Koch (1976a, 1977). He also, like Edwards and Raftery (1976) noted a significant inhibition of the increase in cardiac output during exercise at a work load of about 700kpm/min. The decrease in cardiac output during exercise was due to a reduced heart rate, as stroke volume did not change significantly.

During anaesthesia with 1% halothane, intravenous labetalol 25mg, caused a consistent moderate decrease in cardiac output (5.3l/min to 4.4l/ min), but a marked decrease to 3.51/min occurred when the concentration of halothane was increased to 3% (Scott et al., 1976). This effect was more marked than observed with halothane 3% alone (Scott et al., 1978).

1.2.3 Effect on Peripheral Vascular Resistance

Labetalol, given intravenously or orally consistently lowers peripheral vascular resistance (Joekes and Thompson, 1976; Koch, 1976a, 1977; Mehta and Cohn, 1977; Prichard et al., 1975) although in one study (Edwards and Raftery, 1976) the fall (18%) did not reach a statistically significant level and in another the decrease was insignificant at rest (Koch, 1976a, 1977). The effect of labetalol in decreasing peripheral resistance is in direct contrast to the effect of conventional β-adrenoceptor blocking drugs which cause an initial increase in peripheral resistance, and is compatible with its α-adrenoceptor blocking action. The decrease in peripheral resistance induced by intravenous labetalol 50mg was found by Koch (1976a, 1977) to be greater in the upright position (17%) and during exercise (20%) than in the supine position (11%). Thus, the α-blocking effect was most apparent when sympathetic outflow was greater, on standing and on exercise.

1.3 Effect on Plasma Renin Activity and Plasma Angiotensin II

Oral labetalol 300 to 1,200mg daily given for a few days, produced no significant change in mean plasma renin activity (PRA). Mehta and Cohn (1977) reported a rise in PRA in 4 patients in whom the pretreatment value was low, but PRA fell slightly in the other two patients in whom pretreatment values were high. In 10 patients in whom pretreatment values were compared with those after 8 to 16 months treatment with labetalol (average dosage 1,200mg daily), PRA was significantly reduced (Koch, 1976b). Similarly, Weidman et al. (1978) reported a significant decrease in supine and upright PRA after 2 weeks of treatment with labetalol.

Intravenous labetalol 1 to 2mg/kg significantly lowered plasma angiotensin II in hypertensive patients in whom basal levels were raised. However, in a cross-over study in 5 other patients comparing labetalol 1 to 2mg/kg with propranolol 10mg, only propranolol significantly lowered plasma angiotensin II (Rosei et al., 1976a,b; Trust et al., 1976).

1.4 Effect on Respiratory Function

Although labetalol is non-'cardioselective' in its β-adrenoceptor blocking effects, the presence of its α-adrenoceptor blocking action seems to prevent bronchoconstriction in asthmatic and normal subjects in conditions where ventilatory function might be expected to be lowered.

In a study in asthmatic patients (Skinner et al., 1975), there was no significant change in resting FEV_1 after labetalol 20mg intravenously or placebo, but there was a significant reduction after 5mg of propranolol. There was no significant difference between the treatments with respect to the response to salbutamol 200μg given 1 hour after the drug.

In open studies in hypertensive subjects given intravenous labetalol 1 or 2mg/kg (Pearson and Havard, 1976) or oral labetalol 300, 600 and 1,200mg on consecutive days (Breckenridge et al., 1977a) there was no significant change in peak expiratory flow rate (PEFR). In healthy volunteers, oral propranolol 40 to 160mg produced a greater reduction in PEFR at rest and during exercise than labetalol, the ratio of the effects of the drugs being 14.9:1 at rest and 9.2:1 during exercise (Richards et al., 1977a). Compared with pretreatment values, 80mg propranolol caused a significant reduction in resting FEV_1 before and after histamine inhalation, whilst labetalol and placebo did not.

1.5 Animal Toxicological Studies

Three-month studies with labetalol in dosages of up to 250mg/kg/day orally in the rat and of up to 100mg/kg/day orally in the dog revealed no evidence of drug re-lated toxicity (Poynter et al., 1976). Similarly in chronic studies lasting 1 year, doses of labetalol of up to 200mg/kg in the rat and 100mg/kg in the dog were without toxic effects.

In rats and rabbits given oral labetalol 50 to 200mg/kg/day and in rabbits given 1 to 10mg/kg/day intravenously during pregnancy there was no evidence of adverse effect on the fetus. However, autoradiography of the fetuses of Dutch rabbits given radio-labelled labetalol revealed noticeable radioactivity in the eye (Poynter et al., 1976).

Subsequent study (Poynter et al., 1976) showed that labetalol, but not its meta-bolites, was bound to melanin in the eye and that this binding was reversible. Careful examination of the developing eyes from rabbit fetuses, eyes from weanling rabbits, and the eyes of dogs and cats treated with maximum tolerated dosages for several months, revealed no changes attributable to the drug and suggested that labetalol is continuously bound and released from melanin (Poynter et al., 1976). A study in Dutch rabbits (Poynter et al., 1976) showed that little was bound to the cornea and lens.

1.6 Mode of Action

The mode of action of labetalol in hypertension, like that of the conventional β-adrenoceptor blocking drugs, is not fully known. Although the β-adrenoceptor blocking effect of labetalol is more potent than its α-adrenoceptor blocking effect (Richards et al., 1976a,b,c) and the drug has a greater affinity for β- than the α- adrenoceptor in rat heart and liver (Aggerbeck et al., 1978), the clear reduction in blood pressure produced by intravenous labetalol 2mg/kg in hypertensive patients and in those whose blood pressure was inadequately controlled by β-adrenoceptor blocking drugs, indicates that the α-adrenoceptor blocking effect of labetalol predominates following acute administration of the drug. It is not clear whether α- or β-blocking effects provide the predominant hypotensive effect during longer term oral therapy. The minimal influence of labetalol on heart rate after acute administration may result from its being an inhibitor of postsynaptic function at α-adrenoceptors, thus resembling prazosin.

Dargie et al. (1976) demonstrated that labetalol can lower blood pressure when administered intracisternally in animals, but under normal circumstances and at usual dosages, it is not very likely that labetalol would be present in sufficient concentrations in the central nervous system to produce a predominant central action in man (see section 2.2).

2. Pharmacokinetics

Labetalol is readily absorbed after oral administration, but plasma levels of unchanged drug are low due to considerable first-pass metabolism, bioavailability being about 40% in healthy subjects and 60% in chronic liver disease. About 60% of a dose is excreted in the urine in 24 hours with up to 5% being present as unchanged drug. The major metabolite, a conjugate of labetalol, is without α- or β-adrenoceptor blocking activity in animals.

2.1 Absorption

Labetalol appears to be rapidly absorbed after oral administration in man (Richards et al., 1977c), but plasma levels of the drug itself are low (Breckenridge et al., 1977a; Hopkins et al., 1976; Richards et al., 1977c) and represented only a small proportion (< 5%) of total plasma radioactivity following administration of 3mg/kg of radio-labelled labetalol to 2 adult volunteers (Hopkins et al., 1976; Martin et al., 1976). In a study (Martin et al., 1976) in 5 volunteers given oral doses of 100, 200 and 400mg, plasma concentrations of labetalol were dose related (fig. 3). The ratio of the area under the plasma labetalol-time profile for each of the doses were 1:2.6:5.6 for the 100, 200 and 400mg doses respectively. In patients with chronic liver disease, the area under the plasma concentration-time profile after a single oral dose of 100 or 200mg of labetalol was 3 times that in normal subjects after the same dose (Homeida et al., 1978). Peak plasma concentrations of labetalol are attained 1 to 2 hours after oral administration and vary considerably between individuals (Richards et al., 1977c). Comparison of the area under the plasma concentration versus time curve after intravenous and oral administration of 100 or 200mg to the same subjects indicated a bioavailability of 33 to 40.7% (Breckenridge et al., 1977a; Homeida et al., 1978) but this is increased (Homeida et al., 1978) in patients with chronic liver disease (section 2.5).

2.2 Distribution

Distribution studies in man are few. However, as labetalol is not highly protein bound, it seems likely that in man as in animals (Martin et al., 1976), it is rapidly removed from the plasma and taken up into the tissues after intravenous injection. The volume of distribution in man is large (805 ± 91L), but is significantly decreased in patients with chronic liver disease (526 ± 31L) [Homeida et al., 1978]. Radiochemical analysis of the tissues of rats, rabbits and dogs after injection of labelled drug (Martin et al., 1976) revealed highest concentrations of radioactivity in the lung, liver and kidney. Labetalol is much less lipophilic than propranolol or oxprenolol and there is negligible uptake of labetalol into the brain (Martin et al., 1976). Little radioactivity crossed the placenta and very little of the administered dose of radioactivity entered the fetus of the pregnant rat or rabbit. Labetalol is bound to human plasma protein to the extent of about 50% (Martin et al., 1976).

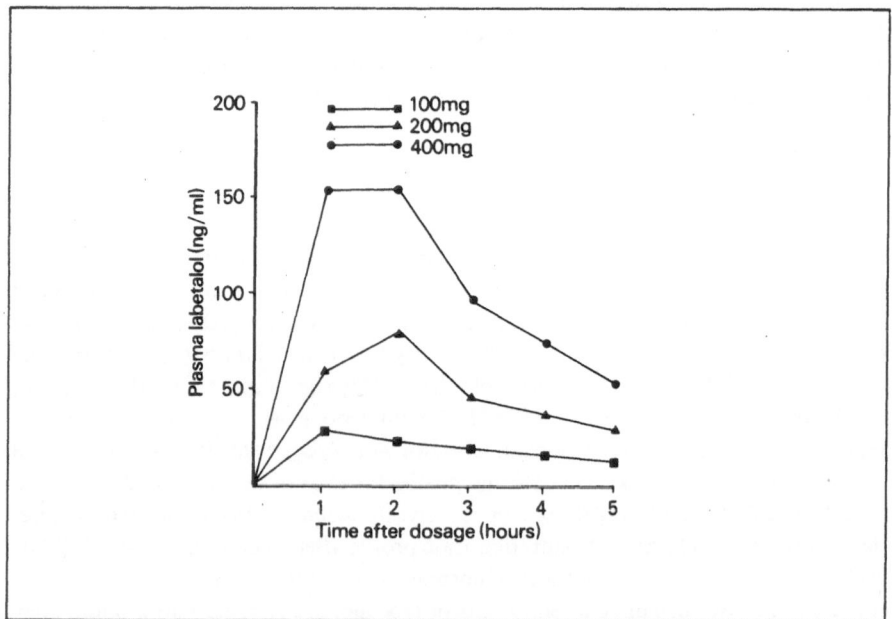

Fig. 3. Mean plasma labetalol concentrations in 5 healthy volunteers given oral doses of 100, 200 and 400mg labetalol (after Martin et al., 1976).

2.3 Elimination

2.3.1 Metabolism

Labetalol is extensively metabolised in man and in animals after oral administration and a study in 5 healthy volunteers recorded 5 % or less of the dose as unchanged drug (Martin et al., 1976). Animal studies suggest that metabolites are formed by first-pass metabolism of labetalol during passage through the intestinal wall and lumen (Martin et al., 1976).

The major metabolite is an unidentified conjugate accounting for 45 % of an oral dose. About 15 % of the dose is present as the o-phenylglucuronide of labetalol (Hopkins et al., 1976; Martin et al., 1976). Neither of these metabolites has exhibited pharmacological activity in animals after oral administration.

2.3.2 Excretion

About 55 to 60 % of an oral dose of labetalol is recovered in the urine of man over a period of 24 hours (Hopkins et al., 1976; Martin et al., 1976). Faecal samples in one subject contained 27.4 % of the administered radioactivity over 96 hours whilst in another subject faecal samples collected for 48 hours contained 12.4 % of the dose administered. Bile concentrations are high in the rabbit (Martin et al., 1976) but data on bile levels in man are not available.

2.3.3 Plasma Half-life

The half-life of elimination of labetalol determined from the terminal portion of the intravenous clearance curve is 3.5 to 4.5 hours in man (Martin et al., 1976). A study (Thompson et al., 1977) in 4 patients with severely impaired renal function showed that the half-life was not altered compared with that reported by others in normal subjects.

2.4 Plasma Concentration and Clinical Effects

A clear relationship between peak plasma concentration of labetalol and maximum pharmacological effect was observed by Richards et al. (1977c) after oral doses of 100, 200 and 400mg. There was a linear correlation (r = 0.84) between the reduction in exercise tachycardia occurring two hours after oral labetalol and the logarithm of the plasma concentration. Similarly, the serial measurements of systolic pressure were closely related to the changing plasma concentration. Fall in heart rate and in diastolic blood pressure was less in normal subjects than in patients with chronic liver disease in whom plasma concentrations were increased after oral labetalol (Homeida et al., 1978). The decline in plasma concentration after oral or intravenous labetalol was steeper than the decline in the pharmacological effects. Similar findings have been reported following single or multiple doses of metoprolol (Regardh et al., 1975) and tolamolol (Faulkner et al., 1975).

2.5 Influence of Disease on Kinetics

In patients with chronic liver disease, the bioavailability of oral labetalol is increased (33 ± 3 to $67 \pm 7\%$) and is inversely related to plasma albumin [Homeida et al., 1978]. In 10 patients with histologically proven liver disease, plasma concentrations after oral labetalol 100 or 200mg (single dose) were considerably higher (section 2.1) than in normal subjects, but were similar in both groups after intravenous administration. Half-life did not differ significantly between patients and normal subjects, but the volume of distribution was significantly smaller in liver disease (section 2.2).

3. Therapeutic Trials

Placebo controlled studies (section 3.2) have shown labetalol to be superior to placebo when given orally in fixed or individually titrated doses to patients with mild, moderate or severe hypertension. Open studies (section 3.1), largely in patients whose blood pressure was not satisfactorily controlled by previous antihypertensive therapy, indicate that labetalol may be particularly useful in some such patients, and a study extending over 3 years suggests that the efficacy of labetalol is comparable with that of α-methyldopa.

Labetalol has been compared, under double-blind conditions, with propranolol and with a combination of oxprenolol and phentolamine (section 3.3). As might be expected titrated doses of labetalol and propranolol produced a similar fall in supine blood pressure, but labetalol produced a greater fall in the upright position. Labetalol 400 and 600mg daily was more effective than oxprenolol 480mg plus phentolamine at a dosage of 60mg daily, which was probably subtherapeutic.

Initial results with intravenous labetalol in the treatment of severe hypertension are promising (section 3.5).

3.1 Open Studies

In open studies, labetalol has been used to treat hypertension largely in patients whose blood pressure was not well controlled by previous treatment (Bolli et al., 1976; Dargie et al., 1976; Jennings and Parsons, 1976) including those with chronic renal failure (Williams et al., 1978), or in patients already receiving other antihypertensive treatment (Morgan et al., 1978; Prichard and Boakes, 1976; Prichard et al., 1975). Open trials reported so far have been conducted over a mean period of at least 5 months and have employed both an arbitrary maximum dosage (Hansson and Hanel, 1976a,b) and dosages which were individually titrated until a desired level of control was achieved or side effects intervened (Bolli et al., 1976; Dargie et al., 1976; Jennings and Parsons, 1976; Prichard and Boakes, 1976).

In previously treated hypertensive patients, Prichard and Boakes (1976) found labetalol 75 to 3,200mg daily (average 889mg) controlled blood pressure to an extent similar to methyldopa in 6 patients, to β-adrenoceptor blocking drugs in 4 patients, and to adrenergic neurone blocking drugs in 7 patients (fig. 4). Although labetalol was not formally compared with these drugs in this study, the study's long term nature (> 3yr in 13 patients) increases the validity of the findings. Prichard and Boakes (1976) reported no change in mean pressure on standing in 26 patients receiving less than 1,800mg labetalol a day, but a fall in mean pressure from 122mm Hg supine, to 111mm Hg standing (p < 0.01) in 4 patients receiving over 1,800mg a day, a significant difference in response from those receiving less than 1,800mg a day (p < 0.002). In the study of Bolli et al. (1976) there was a small fall in blood pressure upon standing with labetalol 200 to 1,200mg daily (mean 585mg) that was absent during previous treatment with the β-adrenoceptor blocking drugs. The postural effect with labetalol was similar to that previously recorded whilst on treatment with various other drugs (fig. 5). However, the postural hypotensive effect was not generally troublesome. Compared with previous therapy, labetalol produced a 17/14mm Hg (mean) fall in supine blood pressure and a 30/20mm Hg fall on standing. A diuretic was given concomitantly with labetalol in all but 1 patient in this study and in all 16 severely hypertensive patients treated by Dargie et al. (1976). These investigators treated resistant patients whose blood pressure was not well controlled by their previous therapy, with labetalol 1,200 to 8,000mg daily (mean

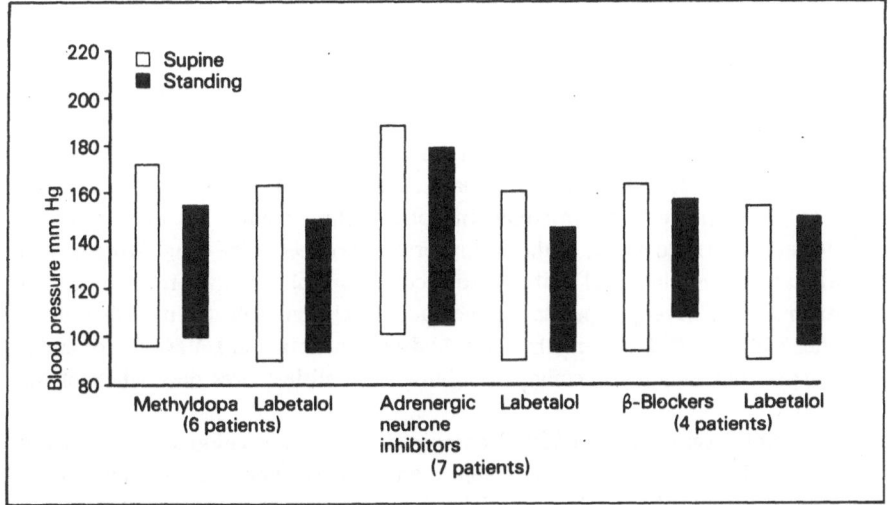

Fig. 4. Mean blood pressure recordings during long term treatment with labetalol 75 to 3,200mg (av 889mg) daily compared with those recorded during previous treatment with α-methyldopa (6 patients), adrenergic neurone blocking drugs (7 patients) or β-adrenoceptor blocking drugs (4 patients) [after Prichard and Boakes, 1976].

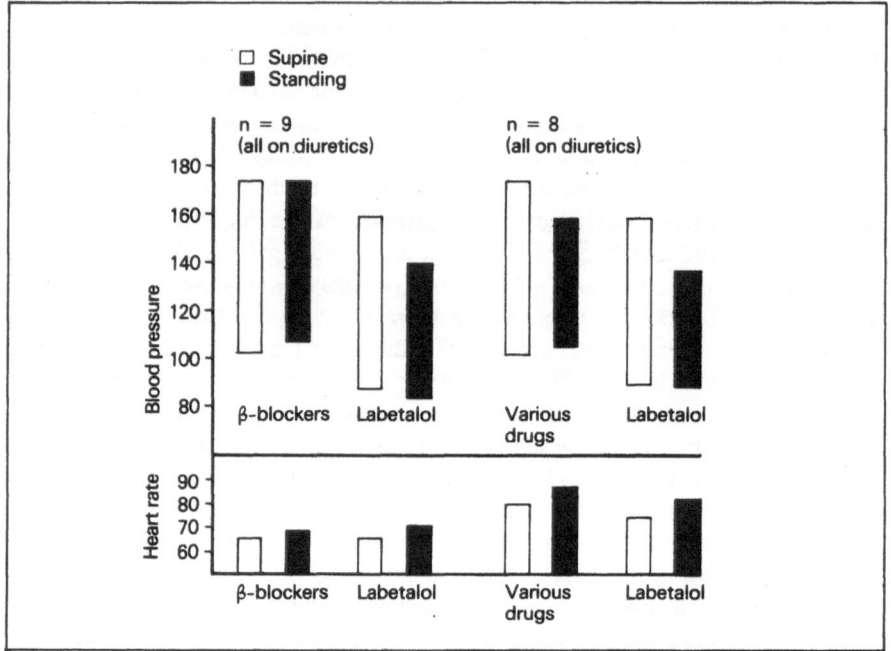

Fig. 5. Mean blood pressure and heart rate recordings on previous antihypertensive therapy which had failed to satisfactorily control blood pressure and after labetalol (200 to 1,200mg; mean 585mg daily) was partly or wholly substituted (after Bolli et al., 1976).

3,091mg), and found that compared with the 6-month period before beginning labetalol, blood pressure improved from 172/108 to 150/98mm Hg in the supine position and from 155/102 to 131/91 in the standing position. Postural effects were reported by some patients during the initial stages of treatment, but these effects were not noted later in the 5-month study. In none of these studies has there been any reported evidence of tolerance to the antihypertensive effect of the drug. Morgan et al. (1978) reported that labetalol enabled satisfactory control of blood pressure in 13 of 22 patients with severe hypertension not adequately controlled with other drugs (diuretic, β-blocker and/or α-methyldopa, hydrallazine, prazosin). Vasodilator and β-adrenoceptor blocking drugs could be withdrawn in all instances once labetalol was established.

Labetalol (average dose 655mg) combined with chlorthalidone 100mg daily, lowered blood pressure to a greater extent than labetalol alone at an average dose of 1,459mg daily in patients with essential hypertension. Orthostatic hypotension occurred less frequently with the combination (Weidman et al., 1978).

An apparent lack of response to the blood pressure lowering effect of labetalol in West Indian and West African patients was reported by Jennings and Parsons (1976) despite dosages of up to 3,200mg daily. There was a statistically significant reduction in blood pressure recorded after 6 months' labetalol treatment in 11 previously untreated and in 26 previously treated Caucasian patients but not in the 10 non-Caucasian patients. There was no significant difference in pulse rate between the three groups. The black patients were heavier than the white patients and their degree of compliance may have been suspect.

In 12 previously untreated patients with mild to moderate essential hypertension (Hansson and Hanel, 1976a,b) labetalol 200 to 600mg daily (average 273mg) significantly reduced mean arterial pressure to the same extent in both supine and standing positions. During the 7-month average period of the study, average supine blood pressure was reduced from 171/109 to 145/83mm Hg.

Labetalol alone (mean dose 913mg daily) or combined with a diuretic, satisfactorily controlled blood pressure in 12 of 18 patients with chronic renal failure with hypertension who were previously treated with multiple drug therapy (13), α-methyldopa (2) or minoxidil (3). Labetalol failed to control blood pressure adequately in the three patients previously controlled on minoxidil (Craswell et al., 1977). Renal function was not adversely affected.

3.2 Placebo Controlled Trials

Placebo controlled trials (table II) in which labetalol has been given in individually titrated doses (Bolli et al., 1976) or fixed doses (Frick and Porsti, 1976; Kane et al., 1976) for periods of 4 to 6 weeks, have demonstrated its superiority to placebo in mild, moderate and severe hypertension. A dose of 300mg labetalol for 4 weeks produced only a slight reduction in blood pressure in the study of Frick and Porsti (1976), but a clinically significant reduction was achieved with 600mg daily. A greater reduction in blood pressure with a dose of 800mg compared with 400mg was reported by Kane et al. (1976) in patients with mild to severe hypertension.

The degree of 'blindness' in the study of Bolli et al. (1976) was questioned by the authors themselves but the possibility of only partial 'blindness' was not raised in the other studies. Labetalol tablets used by Bolli et al. (1976) were described by some patients as 'bitter'.

The postural hypotensive effect evidenced in the study of Bolli et al. (1976) is not apparent in the average figures of Kane et al. (1976), although posture related dizziness was noted. However, in the comparisons with placebo, there is a tendency for a postural effect to be more marked as dosage is increased.

3.3 Labetalol Compared with a β-Adrenoceptor Blocker Alone or in Combination with an α-Adrenoceptor Blocker

A between-patient comparison (Pugsley et al., 1976b) of labetalol and propranolol in 18 previously untreated patients with severe hypertension demon-

Table II. Results of studies comparing labetalol with placebo in the treatment of hypertension

Author	Patient population	Dose (daily)	Duration[1]	Results[2] placebo	labetalol
Bolli et al. (1976)	10 patients who had previously been treated with labetalol	200-1,200mg	6 weeks (diuretic given concomitantly)	183/104 (L) 172/105 (S)	157/93 137/87
Frick and Porsti (1976)	20; 9 untreated; 10 previous therapy discontinued.	300mg	4 weeks	157/102 (L) 156/115 (S)	152/99 145/109
	Diuretic in 1. Mild to moderate hypertension	600mg	4 weeks	159/104 (L) 152/116 (S)	148/97 130/99
Kane et al. (1976)	30 general practice; 24 not previously treated.	400mg	4 weeks	161/101 (Si) 162/103 (S)	141/90 137/90
	Treatment stopped in all but 4 who received diuretics. Mild to severe hypertension	800mg	4 weeks	161/101 (Si) 162/103 (S)	133/83 128/83

1   Duration of treatment with each dose and with placebo.
2   Blood pressure in mm Hg; abbreviations: L = lying; S = standing; Si = sitting.

strated that both drugs gave a similar reduction in supine blood pressure. Labetalol caused a greater reduction than propranolol on standing and after exercise. A diuretic was given for one or two weeks before labetalol or propranolol and continued for the 14 weeks of the comparative trial. Diastolic blood pressure was reduced to below 90mm Hg (supine and standing) in 8 of 9 patients given labetalol and in 5 of 9 given propranolol. Systolic blood pressure was reduced to 130mm Hg or below in all but 1 patient treated with labetalol and in all but 2 patients on propranolol.

The dosage of each drug was increased until a maximum of 2,400mg labetalol or 960mg of propranolol was reached or until standing blood pressure was < 130/85mm Hg, or heart rate was below 48 beats per minute or dose-limiting side effects occurred. Although an optimum dosage ratio for labetalol to propranolol of 2.4:1 was calculated by Pugsley et al. (1976a) in a comparison of both drugs and placebo in patients with mild to moderate hypertension, in the study in severe hypertension (Pugsley et al., 1976b) the dosage ratio was 1.44:1. Mean dosage at the end of the trial was 763mg labetalol and 532mg propranolol.

In a comparison of labetalol and a combination of oxprenolol and phentolamine (Johnson, 1976a,b), labetalol 400mg and 600mg daily reduced supine and standing blood pressure to a significantly greater extent than oxprenolol 480mg plus phentolamine 60mg daily (fig. 6) in the same patients. However, at this dosage, oral phentolamine would be expected to have little therapeutic effect. A combination of pindolol (10 to 20mg twice daily) and hydrallazine in usual therapeutic dosage (50mg 3 times daily), however, produced a fall in blood pressure almost identical to that achieved with labetalol 400 to 800mg twice daily in 14 patients with mild to moderately severe hypertension (Barnett et al., 1978).

3.4 Use in Phaeochromocytoma

Prior to surgical excision of single or multiple phaeochromocytomata adequate control of the effects of catecholamines secreted by the tumour is necessary because of danger to the patient during induction of anaesthesia and when the tumour is manipulated. The usual medical treatment is combined α- and β-adrenoceptor blockade to control the paroxysmal increases in blood pressure in preparation for surgery and to control blood pressure and arrhythmias during surgery.

Rosei et al. (1976c) reported on the successful use of labetalol to control blood pressure in 4 of 5 patients with phaeochromocytoma. In 2 patients labetalol was given initially as an intravenous bolus and treatment was then continued with oral labetalol. In the patient whose blood pressure was not controlled with labetalol (6.4g

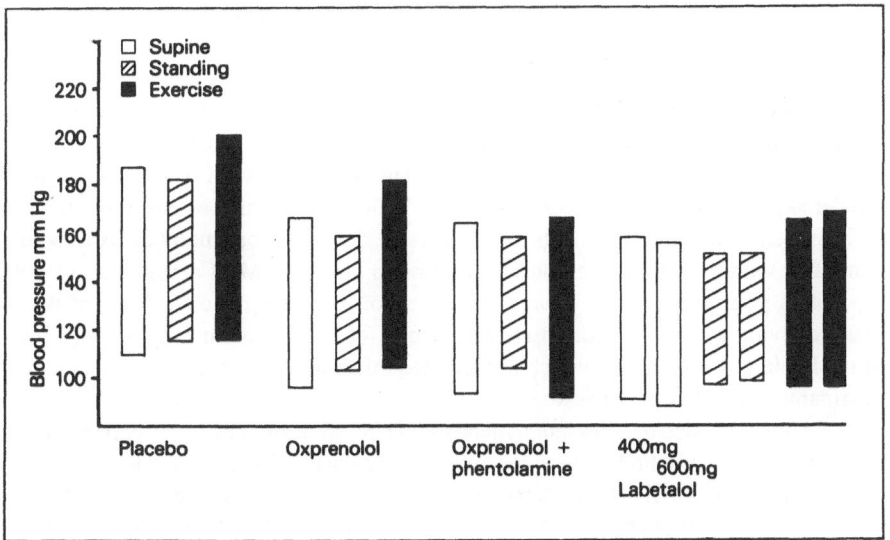

Fig. 6. Mean blood pressure recordings in 13 patients with hypertension during treatment with placebo, oxprenolol 480mg daily alone and combined with phentolamine 60mg daily, and labetalol 400 and 600mg daily (after Johnson et al., 1976a).

daily) blood pressure was well controlled by a combination of phenoxybenzamine and propranolol. Surgical removal of the phaeochromocytomata was successfully conducted under labetalol cover in the 2 patients in whom it was performed.

3.5 Intravenous Labetalol in Severe Hypertension

A prompt fall in systolic and diastolic blood pressure in 20 patients with severe hypertension was produced by the intravenous administration of labetalol 75 to 150mg (1 to 2mg/kg) [Rosei et al., 1976b]. In 16 patients, labetalol was given slowly over 10 minutes, whilst in 4 it was given as a bolus. The fall in blood pressure was well maintained at 3 hours after injection and in 4 patients persisted 18 to 24 hours. The greatest fall was from 188/142mm Hg to 90/64mm Hg 10 minutes after 100mg labetalol.

Although serious hypotension was not observed while the patients were recumbent, hypotension and faintness readily occurred on standing. A satisfactory response in 12 of 18 patients given intravenous labetalol at a dosage of up to 3mg/kg was reported by Wing (1978). Mean arterial blood pressure fell from 219/132 to 145/90mm Hg in those who responded. Each of those who failed to respond showed a satisfactory fall in blood pressure when treated with intravenous diazoxide. Further studies with labetalol given by slow regulated intravenous infusion have been conducted (Brown et al., 1977), but a recent report by Pearson and Harvard (1978) suggested that the magnitude of the fall in blood pressure was the same after fast or slow intravenous injection although the rate of fall can be controlled by varying the rate of injection.

Preliminary experience with intravenous labetalol has been less satisfactory in severely hypertensive patients receiving concomitant therapy with combinations of various other antihypertensive drugs such as β-adrenoceptor blockers, clonidine, α-methyldopa and bethanidine or debrisoquine and in patients with transplant kidneys (Anderson and Gabriel, 1978). Rosei et al. (1976b) reported no response to labetalol in 3 severely hypertensive patients receiving large doses of propranolol or oxprenolol, combined with α-methyldopa and bethanidine in one case. MacCarthy et al. (1978) reported a poor response to intravenous labetalol in 5 of 6 patients. Four of the 5 were receiving additional antihypertensive drugs. The sixth patient experienced a profound fall in blood pressure, which necessitated infusion of a pressor agent to obtain a recordable diastolic blood pressure.

A poor response to intravenous labetalol (1.55 to 3.9mg/kg) in 3 patients with severe hypertension who had received a kidney transplant, was reported by Anderson and Gabriel (1978). All patients were receiving immunosuppressive drugs and 2 were receiving other antihypertensive agents which included propranolol and debrisoquine. In these, as in other patients who had failed to respond to labetalol (vide supra), blood pressure was controlled by intravenous administration of vasodilators (diazoxide, hydrallazine or sodium nitroprusside).

Tachycardia, which accompanied the raised blood pressure in patients with high initial plasma angiotensin II concentrations, was reduced along with the blood pressure and plasma angiotensin II concentration after labetalol administration (Rosei et al., 1976b).

3.6 Labetalol in Clonidine Withdrawal Hypertension

The successful use of labetalol 150mg intravenously to control a severe increase in blood pressure (232/170mm Hg) probably resulting from the abrupt withdrawal of clonidine, has been described by Rosei et al. (1976c). Blood pressure had been poorly controlled with a combination of antihypertensive agents before the withdrawal of clonidine.

4. What is the Role of Labetalol in Hypertension?

Labetalol has been demonstrated to possess both α- and β-adrenoceptor blocking effects in normal and hypertensive persons (section 1.1) and has been shown in therapeutic trials, well designed though limited in number, to be generally effective in reducing blood pressure in mild to moderate hypertension and also in many patients with severe hypertension. Like conventional β-adrenoceptor blocking drugs continuous treatment with labetalol reduces pulse rate, but this effect tends to be less marked than that with doses of conventional β-adrenoceptor blocking agents required to produce a similar reduction in blood pressure.

As labetalol has α-blocking properties in addition to a β-blocking effect, it theoretically offers some advantages over 'pure' β-adrenoceptor blocking drugs in the treatment of hypertension. However, the long term advantage of labetalol over drugs with β-blocking properties alone has yet to be conclusively demonstrated. Inherent in its α-adrenoceptor blocking effect is the tendency to cause on occasions failure of ejaculation and nasal stuffiness, but not the disabling effects which may accompany the use of effective hypotensive dosages of phenoxybenzamine.

As might be expected on theoretical grounds, the α-adrenoceptor blocking effect of labetalol results in a degree of postural hypotension which is more apparent at higher dose levels above about 800mg daily orally. The postural hypotensive effect is quite marked after intravenous administration. Although some authors have stated that postural hypotension has not proved to be a major problem (e.g. Bolli et al., 1976; Breckenridge et al., 1977b) labetalol has yet to be shown in therapeutic trials to have any advantage over conventional β-adrenoceptor blocking drugs in the routine treatment of mild to moderate hypertension.

However, labetalol may have some advantage in that it produces less deviation of haemodynamics from normal after acute administration.

Therapeutic studies (section 3.1) indicate that labetalol may be effective, particularly in the upright position, in many patients whose blood pressure is not adequately controlled by β-adrenoceptors alone, but it is not known if the postural effect is desirable.

As with conventional β-adrenoceptor blocking drugs, patients do not become tolerant to the hypotensive effect of labetalol, blood pressure control being well maintained without the necessity of increasing the dose. Nevertheless, labetalol may cause an increase in plasma and blood volume (Weidman et al., 1978) which may reduce the sensitivity of supine blood pressure to treatment. This effect can be avoided with concomitant diuretic therapy.

Labetalol has been shown to be less likely than propranolol to cause bronchoconstriction in asthmatic patients (section 1.4), but it has not been compared with the 'cardioselective' β-adrenoceptor blockers and it would seem unwise to use labetalol in asthmatic subjects on the basis of present published evidence. The α-adrenoceptor blocking effect of labetalol may impart some advantage in patients who experience Raynaud's phenomenon on conventional β-adrenoceptor blocking drugs (Bolli et al., 1978).

Labetalol looks promising as an intravenous agent in severe hypertension, but further study to determine the best method of administration and optimum dosage is necessary before it can be used routinely for the occasional patient requiring intravenous antihypertensive therapy.

5. Side Effects

The most troublesome side effect reported during oral labetalol therapy is posture related dizziness which occurs in about 5% of patients after 4 weeks' treatment with 300mg daily (Robertson, personal communication). In some instances it has been associated with documented postural hypotension and has occasionally necessitated withdrawal of labetalol. An exaggerated response to the first dose has been reported in 2 patients (Louis et al., 1978). Postural effects tend to occur more frequently with higher dosages (Kane et al., 1976; Dargie et al., 1976) than with low dosages (Hansson and Hanel, 1976) and early in the course of treatment (Dargie et al., 1976) and may be less prominent in patients not taking a diuretic (Bolli et al., 1978), although this was not the experience of Weidman et al. (1978).

Side effects generally, appear to be more frequent during the first few weeks of treatment than later in the course (Pugsley et al., 1976b).

Other side effects which may occur occasionally include tiredness and weakness, muscle cramps, mild constipation, gastrointestinal discomfort, skin rash, headache, nausea, abdominal pain, vivid dreams (1 case) [Hansson and Hanel, 1976; Pugsley et al., 1976b], mental depression (1 case), failure of ejaculation, and scalp tingling (Hua et al., 1977; Frick and Porsti, 1976; Scowen, 1978) — which has also been reported after intravenous therapy (Collier et al., 1972; Bailey, 1977; Wing, 1978), and lichenoid eruptions (Grange and Jones, 1978; Savage et al., 1978). A pressor response has been reported after intravenous (Crofton and Gabriel, 1977; Wing, 1978) and after oral (Briggs et al., 1978) labetalol in a patient with phaeochromocytoma. Intravenous hydrallazine produced a prompt and sustained fall in blood pressure in the patient reported by Crofton and Gabriel (1977).

Positive antinuclear factor (ANF) has been reported occasionally (Bolli et al., 1976; Louis et al., 1978; Pugsley et al., 1976b; Savage et al., 1978) but the significance of these findings is not clear and the effect is not positively associated with labetalol.

Increased angina pectoris in a patient in whom labetalol was substituted for metoprolol, was reported by Bolli et al. (1976) and may simply indicate that labetalol was less effective than metoprolol in controlling the angina.

There have been no reports of ophthalmological effects related to labetalol, and in some studies (Bolli et al., 1976; Hansson and Hanel, 1976; Jennings and Parsons, 1976) eye toxicity has specifically been stated as being absent after suitable investigation.

6. Precautions

As with conventional β-adrenoceptor blocking drugs heart failure should be controlled with digitalis and diuretic therapy before labetalol is administered.

Until further information is available on the effects of labetalol on respiratory function in asthmatics, the drug, like other drugs with β-adrenoceptor blocking activity, is best avoided where possible in patients with asthma.

Patients receiving labetalol who require general anaesthesia should be given intravenous atropine before induction to minimise bradycardia. The effect of halothane on blood pressure may be enhanced by labetalol.

It is probably wise to use labetalol with caution in patients with intermittent claudication, as symptoms can be worsened when arterial pressure is lowered. As the bioavailability of oral labetalol is considerably increased in patients with chronic liver disease, their oral dosage requirements may be lower than in patients without liver disease (section 2.5).

7. Dosage

7.1 Initial Dosage, Oral

The starting dose is 100mg twice or three times daily preferably after food. This dosage may be sufficient to control blood pressure in some patients with mild hypertension, particularly when a diuretic is given concomitantly, but higher dosages are usually necessary for optimum response. However, some patients with severe hypertension may respond to quite small doses.

7.2 Dosage Adjustment

If the reduction in blood pressure is less than optimal after one or two weeks, the dose should be increased to 200mg three or four times daily. In severe cases, under close supervision, dosage can be increased more quickly. The effective dose of labetalol is usually 300 to 800mg in mild to moderate hypertension, 600 to 1,200mg in moderately severe hypertension and 1,200 to 2,400mg daily in severe hypertension. Doses lower than these may be adequate in patients who are also receiving a diuretic.

In patients with angina pectoris, concomitant therapy with conventional β-adrenoceptor blocking drugs may be needed to control the angina.

7.3 Intravenous Labetalol

Intravenous labetalol is indicated for use in hospitalised patents in whom rapid control of severe hypertension is necessary. Patients should always be supine when given labetalol intravenously and should not be raised into the upright position for 3 hours after administration. The drug may be given by bolus injection or by intravenous infusion. A satisfactory response may be obtained less often in patients receiving concomitant therapy with β-adrenoceptor blocking and other antihypertensive drugs.

If given by bolus injection a dose of 50mg should be given over a period of 1 minute. If necessary, doses of 50mg may be repeated at 5-minute intervals until a satisfactory response occurs. The total dose should generally not exceed 200mg. After bolus injection the maximum effect usually occurs within 5 minutes and usually lasts about 6 hours.

If given by infusion, a solution should be made by diluting 200mg labetalol (40ml) to 200ml with sodium chloride and dextrose injection BP. The rate of infusion should be about 2mg (2ml of infusion solution) per minute, until a satisfactory response is obtained; the infusion should then be stopped. The effective dose range is usually 50 to 200mg but doses of 300mg or greater may be needed in patients with phaeochromocytoma. Blood pressure, and preferably also pulse rate, should be monitored throughout the infusion.

Once the blood pressure has been adequately reduced, maintenance therapy with oral labetalol should be initiated.

Acknowledgements

This manuscript was reviewed by: *R.W. Gifford*, The Cleveland Clinic Foundation, Cleveland, Ohio, USA; *P. Kincaid-Smith*, University of Melbourne, Royal Melbourne Hospital, Victoria, Australia; *G. Koch*, Centrallasarettet, Karlskrona, West Germany; *J.G. Ledingham*, University of Oxford, Oxford, England; *B.N.C. Prichard*, University College Hospital Medical School, London, England; *J.I.S. Robertson*, MRC Blood Pressure Unit, Glasgow, Scotland; *F.O. Simpson*, Wellcome Medical Research Institute, University of Otago, Dunedin, New Zealand; *G.S. Stokes*, Kanematsu Memorial Institute, Sydney Hospital, Sydney, Australia.

References

Aggerbeck, M.; Guellaen, G. and Hanoure, J.: Biochemical evidence for the dual action of labetalol on α- and β-adrenoceptors. British Journal of Pharmacology 62: 543 (1978).

Anderson, C.C. and Gabriel, R.: Poor hypotensive response and tachyphylaxis following intravenous labetalol. Current Medical Research and Opinion 5: 424 (1978).

Andersson, O.; Berglund, G. and Hansson, L.: Antihypertensive action, time of onset and effects on carbohydrate metabolism of labetalol. British Journal of Clinical Pharmacology 3 (Suppl.): 757 (1976).

Bailey, R.R.: Scalp tingling and difficulty in micturition in patients on labetalol. Lancet 2: 720 (1977).

Barnett, A.J.; Kalowski, S. and Guest, C.: Labetalol compared with pindolol plus hydrallazine in the treatment of hypertension. Medical Journal of Australia 1: 105 (1978).

Blakeley, A.G.H. and Summers, R.J.: The effects of AH 5158 on the overflow of transmitter and the uptake of [³H]-(-)-noradrenaline in the cat spleen. British Journal of Pharmacology 56: 364P (1976).

Blakeley, A.G.H. and Summers, R.J.: The effects of labetalol (AH 5158) on adrenergic transmission in the cat spleen. British Journal of Pharmacology 59: 643 (1977).

Bolli, P.; Waal-Manning, H.J.; Wood, A.J. and Simpson, F.O.: Experience with labetalol in hypertension. British Journal of Clinical Pharmacology 3 (Suppl.): 765 (1976).

Bolli, P.; Waal-Manning, H.J.; Simpson, F.O. and Seeman, H.M.I.: Treatment of hypertension with labetalol, a new antihypertensive drug which combines α- and β-adrenoceptor blockade. New Zealand Medical Journal: in press (1978).

Breckenridge, A.M.; Macnee, C.M.; Orme, M.L'E.; Richards, D.A. and Sterlin, M.J.: Rate of onset of hypotensive response with oral labetalol. British Journal of Clinical Pharmacology 4: 338P (1977a).

Breckenridge, A.; Calvey, T.N.; Green, G.J.; McIver, M.; Orme, M.L'E. and Serlin, M.J.: Labetalol in hypertension. Lancet 2: 36 (1977b).

Briggs, R.S.J.; Birtwell, A.J. and Pohl, J.E.F.: Hypertensive response to labetalol in phaeochromocytoma. Lancet 1: 1045 (1978).

Brittain, R.T. and Levy, G.P.: A review of the animal pharmacology of labetalol, a combined α- and β-adrenoceptor blocking drug. British Journal of Clinical Pharmacology 3 (Suppl.): 681 (1976).

Brown, J.J.; Lever, A.F.; Cumming, A.M.M. and Robertson, J.I.S.: Labetalol in hypertension. Lancet 1: 1147 (1977).

Cambridge, D.; Davey, M.J. and Massingham, R.: Prazosin, a selective antagonist of post-synaptic α-adrenoceptors. British Journal of Pharmacology 59: 514P (1977).

Collier, J.G.; Dawnay, N.A.H.; Nachev, C.H. and Robinson, B.F.: Clinical investigation of an antagonist at α- and β-adrenoceptors — AH 5158A. British Journal of Pharmacology 44: 286 (1972).

Craswell, P.; Williams, J. and de Voss, K.: Labetalol in chronic renal failure with hypertension. Australian and New Zealand Journal of Medicine 7: 441 (1977).

Crofton, M. and Gabriel, R.: Pressor response after intravenous labetalol. British Medical Journal 2: 737 (1977).

Dargie, H.J.; Dollery, C.T. and Daniel, J.: Labetalol in resistant hypertension. British Journal of Clinical
    Pharmacology 3 (Suppl.): 751 (1976).
Edwards, R.C. and Raftery, E.B.: Haemodynamic effects of long-term oral labetalol. British Journal of
    Clinical Pharmacology 3 (Suppl.): 733 (1976).
Farmer, J.B.; Kennedy, I.; Levy, G.P. and Marshall, R.J.: Pharmacology of AH 5158; a drug which
    blocks both α- and β-adrenoceptors. British Journal of Pharmacology 45: 660 (1972).
Faulkner, J.K.; Stopher, D.A.; Walden, R.; Singleton, W. and Taylor, W.: Pharmacokinetic and pharma-
    cological studies with tolamolol in man. British Journal of Clinical Pharmacology 2: 423 (1975).
Frick, M.H. and Porsti, P.: Combined alpha- and beta-adrenoceptor blockade with labetalol in hyperten-
    sion. British Medical Journal 1: 1046 (1976).
Grange, R.W. and Jones, E.W.: Bullous lichen planus caused by labetalol. British Medical Journal 1: 816
    (1978).
Hansson, L. and Hanel, B.: Labetalol, a new α- and β-adrenoceptor blocking agent in hypertension. Bri-
    tish Journal of Clinical Pharmacology 3 (Suppl.): 763 (1976a).
Hansson, L. and Hanel, B.: Antihypertensive effect of labetalol, a new alpha- and beta-adrenergic block-
    ing agent. International Journal of Clinical Pharmacology 14: 195 (1976b).
Harichaux, P. and Hary, L.: Some complementary data on AH 5158, an inhibitor of both α- and β-
    adrenoceptors. British Journal of Pharmacology 58: 412P (1976).
Homeida, M.; Jackson, L. and Roberts, C.J.C.: Decreased first-pass metabolism of labetalol in chronic
    liver disease. Britsh Medical Journal 2: 1048 (1978).
Hopkins, R.; Martin, L.E. and Bland, R.: The metabolism of labetalol in animals and man. Biochemical
    Society Transactions 4: 726 (1976).
Hua, A.S.P.; Thomas, G.W. and Kincaid-Smith, P.: Scalp tingling in patients on labetalol. Lancet 2: 295
    (1977).
Jennings, K. and Parsons, V.: A study of labetalol in patients of European, West Indian and West African
    origin. British Journal of Clinical Pharmacology 3 (Suppl): 773 (1976).
Joekes, A.M. and Thompson, F.D.: Acute haemodynamic effects of labetalol and its subsequent use as an
    oral hypotensive agent. British Journal of Clinical Pharmacology 3 (Suppl): 789 (1976).
Johnson, B.F.; La Brooy, J. and Munro-Faure, A.D.: The anti-hypertensive efficacy of combined α- and
    β-adrenoceptor blockade with phentolamine-oxprenolol or with labetalol (AH 5158). Clinical
    Science and Molecular Medicine 51: 505s (1976a).
Johnson, B.F.; La Brooy, J. and Munro-Faure, A.D.: Comparative anti-hypertensive effects of labetalol
    and the combination of oxprenolol and phentolamine. British Journal of Clinical Pharmacology 3
    (Suppl): 783 (1976b).
Kane, J.; Gregg, I. and Richards, D.A.: A double-blind trial of labetalol. British Journal of Clinical Phar-
    macology 3 (Suppl): 737 (1976).
Kennedy, I. and Levy, G.P.: Combined α- and β-adrenoceptor blocking drug AH 5158: Further studies
    on α-adrenoceptor blocking drug blockade in anaesthetised animals. British Journal of Pharma-
    cology 53: 585 (1975).
Koch, G.: Haemodynamic effects of combined α- and β-adrenoceptor blockade after intravenous labetalol
    in hypertensive patients at rest and during exercise. British Journal of Clinical Pharmacology 3 (Sup-
    pl): 725 (1976a).
Koch, G.: Combined α- and β-adrenoceptor blockade with oral labetalol in hypertensive patients with
    reference to haemodynamic effects at rest and during exercise. British Journal of Clinical Pharma-
    cology 3 (Suppl): 729 (1976b).
Koch, G.: Acute hemodynamic effects of an alpha- and beta-receptor blocking agent (AH 5158) on the
    systemic and pulmonary circulation at rest and during exercise in hypertensive patients. American
    Heart Journal 93: 585 (1977).
Louis, W.J.; Brignell, M.J.; McNeil, J.J.; Christopher, N. and Vajda, F.J.E.: Labetalol in hypertension.
    Lancet 1: 452 (1978).

Maconochie, J.G.; Richards, D.A. and Woodings, E.P.: Modification of pressor responses induced by 'cold'. British Journal of Clinical Pharmacology 4: 389P (1977a).

Maconochie, J.G.; Woodings, E.P. and Richards, D.A.: Effects of labetalol and propranolol on histamine-induced bronchoconstriction in normal subjects. British Journal of Clinical Pharmacology 4: 157 (1977b).

MacCarthy, E.P.; Frost, G.W. and Stokes, G.S.: Labetalol in hypertensive emergencies: Medical Journal of Australia 1: 399 (1978).

Martin, L.E.; Hopkins, R. and Bland, R.: Metabolism of labetalol by animals and man. British Journal of Clinical Pharmacology 3 (Suppl): 695 (1976).

Maxwell, G.M.: The effects of a new α- and β-adrenoceptor antagonist (AH 5158) upon the general and coronary haemodynamics of intact dogs. British Journal of Pharmacology 42: 370 (1973).

Mehta, J. and Cohn, J.N.: Hemodynamic effects of labetalol, an alpha and beta adrenergic blocking agent, in hypertensive subjects. Circulation 55: 370 (1977).

Morgan, T.; Gillies, A.; Morgan. G. and Adam, W.: The effect of labetalol in the treatment of severe drug-resistant hypertension. Medical Journal of Australia 1: 393 (1978).

Pearson, R.M. and Havard, C.W.H.: Intravenous labetalol in hypertensive patients treated with β-adrenoceptor blocking drugs. British Journal of Clinical Pharmacology 3 (Suppl): 795 (1976).

Pearson, R.M. and Havard, C.W.H.: Intravenous labetalol in hypertensive patients given by fast and slow injection. British Journal of Clinical Pharmacology 5: 401 (1978).

Poynter, D.; Martin, L.E.; Harrison, C. and Cook, J.: Affinity of labetalol for ocular melanin. British Journal of Clinical Pharmacology 3 (Suppl): 711 (1976).

Prichard, B.N.C. and Boakes, A.J.: Labetalol in long-term treatment of hypertension. British Journal of Clinical Pharmacology 3 (Suppl): 743 (1976).

Prichard, B.N.C.; Thompson, F.O.; Boakes, A.J. and Joekes, A.M.: Some haemodynamic effects of compound AH 5158 compared with propranolol, propranolol plus hydrallazine, and diazoxide: the use of AH 5158 in the treatment of hypertension. Clinical Science and Molecular Medicine 48: 97s (1975).

Pugsley, D.; Armstrong, B.; Nassim, M. and Beilin, L.J.: Combined α- and β-adrenoreceptor blockade in hypertension: a controlled trial of labetalol (AH 5158) compared with propranolol and placebo. Clinical Science and Molecular Medicine 51: 501s (1976a).

Pugsley, D.J.; Armstrong, B.K.; Nassim, M.A. and Beilin, L.J.: Controlled comparison of labetalol and propranolol in the management of severe hypertension. British Journal of Clinical Pharmacology 3 (Suppl): 777 (1976b).

Regardh, C.-G.; Johnsson, G.; Jordo, L. and Solvell, L.: Comparative bioavailability and effect studies on metoprolol administered as ordinary and slow-release tablets in single and multiple doses. Acta Pharmacologica et Toxicologica 36 (Suppl. V): 45 (1975).

Richards, D.A. and Prichard, B.N.C.: Concurrent antagonism of isoprenaline and noradrenaline after labetalol in man. Clinical Pharmacology and Therapeutics: 23: 253 (1978).

Richards, D.A.; Maconochie, J.G.; Bland, R.E.; Hopkins, R.; Woodings, E.P. and Martin, L.E.: Relationship between plasma concentrations and pharmacological effects of labetalol. European Journal of Clinical Pharmacology 11: 85 (1977c).

Richards, D.A.; Prichard, B.N.C.; Boakes, A.J.; Tuckman, J. and Knight, E.J.: Pharmacological basis for antihypertensive effects of intravenous labetalol. British Heart Journal 39: 99 (1977b).

Richards, D.A.; Tuckman, J. and Prichard, B.N.C.: Assessment of α- and β-adrenoceptor blocking actions of labetalol. British Journal of Clinical Pharmacology 3: 849 (1976a).

Richards, D.A.; Tuckman, J. and Prichard, B.N.C.: Combined α- and β-adrenoceptor blockade with labetalol at rest and during exercise. British Journal of Clinical Pharmacology 3: 967P (1976b).

Richards, D.A.; Tuckman, J. and Prichard, B.N.C.: Assessment of the α- and β-adrenoceptor blocking properties of labetalol (AH 5158) after oral administration to normal volunteers. British Journal of Clinical Pharmacology 3: 343P (1976c).

Richards, D.A.; Woodings, E.P. and Maconochie, J.G.: Comparison of the effects of labetalol and propranolol in healthy men at rest and during exercise. British Journal of Clinical Pharmacology 4: 15 (1977a).

Richards, D.A.; Woodings, E.P.; Stephens, M.D.B. and Maconochie, J.G.: The effects of oral AH 5158, a combined α- and β-adrenoceptor antagonist, in healthy volunteers. British Journal of Clinical Pharmacology 1: 505 (1974).

Rønne-Rasmussen, J.O.; Andersen, G.S.; Bowal Jensen, N. and Andersson, E.: Acute effect of intravenous labetalol in the treatment of systemic arterial hypertension. British Journal of Clinical Pharmacology 3 (Suppl): 805 (1976).

Rosei, E.A.; Trust, P.M.; Brown, J.J.; Fraser, R.; Lever, A.F.; Morton, J.J. and Robertson, J.I.S.: Effects of intravenous labetalol on blood pressure, angiotensin II and aldosterone in hypertension: comparison with propranolol. Clinical Science and Molecular Medicine 51: 497s (1976a).

Rosei, E.A.; Brown, J.J.; Fraser, R.; Lever, A.F.; Morton, J.J.; Robertson, J.I.S. and Trust, P.M.: Labetalol (AH 5158), a competitive alpha- and beta-receptor blocking drug, in the management of hypertension. Australia and New Zealand Journal of Medicine 6 (Suppl. 3): 83 (1976b).

Rosei, E.A.; Brown, J.J.; Lever, A.F.; Robertson, A.S.; Robertson, J.I.S. and Trust, R.M.: Treatment of phaeochromocytoma and of clonidine withdrawal hypertension with labetalol. British Journal of Clinical Pharmacology 3 (Suppl): 809 (1976c).

Savage, R.L.; Lesna, M.; Mucklow, J.C. and Stevenson, C.J.: Cutaneous reactions to labetalol. British Medical Journal 1: 987 (1978).

Scott, D.B.; Buckley, F.P.; Drummond, G.B.; Littlewood, D.G. and Macrae, W.R.: Cardiovascular effects of labetalol during halothane anaesthesia. British Journal of Clinical Pharmacology 3 (Suppl): 817 (1976).

Scott, D.B.; Buckley, F.P.; Littlewood, D.G.; Macrae, W.R.; Arthur, G.R. and Drummond, G.B.: Circulatory effects of labetalol during halothane anaesthesia. Anaesthesia 33: 145 (1978).

Scowen, E.: Scalp tingling on labetalol. Lancet 1: 98 (1978).

Skinner, C.; Gaddie, J. and Palmer, K.N.V.: Comparison of intravenous AH 5158 (ibidomide) and propranolol in asthma. British Medical Journal 2: 59 (1975).

Thompson, F.D.; Joekes, A.M. and Hussein, M.M.: Labetalol used as a hypotensive agent in the presence of renal disease. Kidney International Journal 11: 287 (1977).

Trust, P.M.; Rosei, E.A.; Brown, J.J.; Fraser, R.; Lever, A.F.; Morton, J.J. and Robertson, J.I.S.: Effect on blood pressure, angiotensin II and aldosterone concentrations during treatment of severe hypertension with intravenous labetalol: comparison with propranolol. British Journal of Clinical Pharmacology 3 (Suppl): 799 (1976).

Weidman, P.; De Chatel, R.; Ziegler, W.H.; Flammer, J. and Reubi, F.: Alpha and beta adrenergic blockade with orally administered labetalol in hypertension. Studies on blood volume, plasma renin and aldosterone and catecholamine excretion. American Journal of Cardiology 41: 570 (1978).

Williams, J.G.; De Voss, K. and Craswell, P.W.; Labetalol in the treatment of hypertensive renal patients. Medical Journal of Australia 1: 225 (1978)

Wing, L.M.H.: Labetalol in hypertensive emergencies. Medical Journal of Australia 1: 659 (1978).

Chapter IV

Prazosin: A Review of its Pharmacological Properties and Therapeutic Efficacy

R.N. Brogden, R.C. Heel, T.M. Speight and G.S. Avery

1. Animal Pharmacodynamic Studies

1.1 Mode of Action

Prazosin [1-(4-amino-6,7-dimethoxy-2-quinazolinyl)-4-(2-furoyl)-piperazine] is the first member of a new class of antihypertensive agents (fig. 1).

Prazosin appears to exert its antihypertensive effect by relaxation of peripheral arterioles as a consequence of functional blockade of postsynaptic α-adrenoceptors, rather than by a direct relaxation of arteriolar vascular muscle. It differs from other α-adrenoceptor blocking drugs such as phentolamine, which act at pre- as well as postsynaptic α-adrenoceptors, and from diazoxide and hydrallazine which lower blood pressure by a direct action on vascular smooth muscle. However, prazosin resembles diazoxide in acting primarily on arterioles rather than arteries.

Although the work of Constantine (1974) suggested that the hypotensive effect of prazosin is due to two components of vasodilator action, namely atypical α-adrenoceptor blockade and direct relaxation of arteriolar smooth muscle, findings of several recent studies are compatible with a sympatholytic mode of action (Cavero, 1976; Cavero and Lefevre, 1976; Cavero et al., 1977a; Graham et al., 1976a; Jauernig and Moulds, 1976; Jauernig et al, 1978; Scivoletto et al., 1976; Simpson, 1977). Recent evidence confirms that prazosin exerts its hypotensive effects by α-adrenoceptor blockade and not by a *direct* smooth muscle relaxant effect (Oates et al., 1976, 1977; Cavero and Lefevre, 1976; Graham et al., 1977; Stokes and Oates, 1977). The nature of the α-adrenoceptor occupancy is different from that of phenoxybenzamine (Cambridge et al., 1977b) and it has been demonstrated by Massingham et al. (1977)

that prazosin has an affinity for postsynaptic α-adrenoceptors, but little or no affinity
for presynaptic α-adrenoceptors. Unlike α-methyldopa and clonidine, prazosin appears to have no central action on blood pressure (Cambridge et al., 1976b; Wood et
al., 1975).

Experiments in animals indicate that prazosin 0.1mg/kg/min reduces peripheral vascular resistance (Constantine et al., 1973) and that this effect depends upon
intact sympathetic innervation (Cavero and Lefevre, 1976; Cavero et al., 1978;
Simpson, 1977; Wood et al., 1975). Dog forelimb studies (Constantine et al., 1973)
indicated that 91 % of the reduction in total paw resistance occurred in small vessels
and 7 % in arteries. Venous resistance was not affected (table I). In this regard
prazosin resembles diazoxide, but differs from sodium nitrite and phentolamine, both
of which caused considerable reduction in large-vessel as well as small-vessel resistance. On the other hand, prazosin resembles phentolamine and differs from diazoxide in the manner in which it achieves peripheral vasodilatation. Like phentolamine it
has been shown to cause reversal of adrenaline induced pressor responses in animals
(an effect normally regarded as proof of α-adrenoceptor blockade) [Constantine et
al., 1973; Oates et al., 1977; Stokes and Oates, 1977], but unlike diazoxide it has no
effect on angiotensin induced pressor responses (Oates et al., 1977; Stokes and Oates,
1977).

The finding that the hypotensive effect of prazosin was not affected significantly
by pretreatment with atropine, propranolol, timolol (Oates et al., 1976), tripelen-
namine or sodium nitrite, indicates that the peripheral dilatation effect is not mediated
by endogenous acetylcholine, histamine or a drug interaction with β-adrenoceptors
(Constantine et al., 1973). Equal reduction of nictitating membrane contractions induced by electrical stimulation of pre- or postganglionic fibres of the superior cervical
ganglion suggests that prazosin has no conventional hexamethonium-like ganglionic
blocking activity. Also the absence of any initial pressor response after intravenous
injection and the lack of potentiation of the effects of exogenous catecholamines (Constantine, 1974; Wood et al., 1975) or of dimethylphenylpiperazine, indicate that the
drug does not act by neuronal adrenergic blockade (Constantine et al., 1973). A ten-

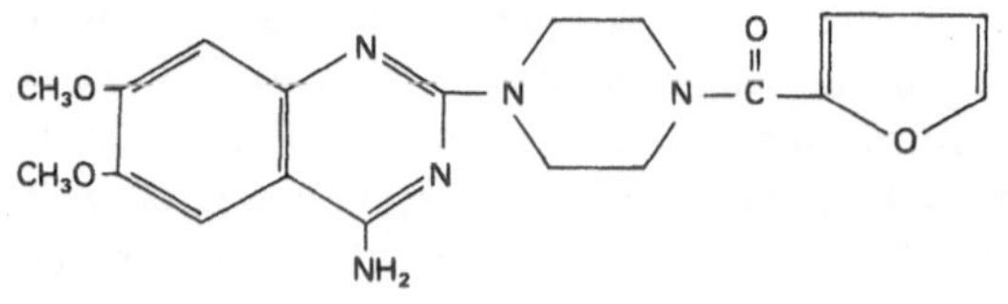

Fig. 1. Structural formula of prazosin.

Table I. Pattern of distribution of vascular resistance changes of 4 peripheral vasodilator compounds in the perfused dog forelimb (after Constantine et al., 1973)

Drug	Dose (intra-arterial mg/ml/min)	Percentage decrease in paw resistance		
		small vessels	paw arteries	paw veins
Prazosin	0.1	91 ± 8	7 ± 1	2 ± 2
Diazoxide	0.5	93 ± 2	7 ± 0.4	0
Sodium nitrite	0.5	74 ± 6	24 ± 2	2 ± 0.4
Phentolamine	0.01	68 ± 4	29 ± 3	3 ± 2

dency for baroreceptor sensitivity to increase in cats after prazosin administration ($40\mu g/kg$ i.v.) was noted by Cambridge et al. (1977b). This effect was also exhibited by intravenous hydrallazine ($2mg/kg$) and minoxidil ($2mg/kg$).

Recent evidence indicates that prazosin produces a reduction in blood pressure by blocking α-adrenoceptors (*vide supra*). However, unlike conventional α-adrenoceptor blocking agents prazosin did not cause tachycardia or renin release in dogs (Constantine, 1974; Massingham and Hayden, 1975). A study by Cambridge et al., (1977a,b) demonstrated that prazosin has a specificity for postsynaptic α-adrenoceptors with little or no affinity for presynaptic receptors *in vitro*. This has been confirmed *in vivo* in rats (Cavero et al., 1977; Hua and Moulds, 1977; Roach et al., 1978). However, prazosin inhibited both pre- and postsynaptic α-adrenoceptors in the dog (Cavero et al., 1977; Roach et al., 1978) and cat (Roach et al., 1978). The specificity for postsynaptic α-receptors probably accounts for the absence of tachycardia and renin release, as it has been postulated that transmitter noradrenaline regulates its own release through a negative feedback mechanism mediated by presynaptic α-receptors (Rand et al., 1975). Thus, blockade of pre- (as well as post-) synaptic α-adrenoceptors by conventional α-blocking drugs causes a loss of the feedback inhibitory mechanism with consequent enhancement of noradrenaline release. Unlike phenoxybenzamine, prazosin, in concentrations which produced similar antagonism of postsynaptic events, did not cause increased noradrenaline release in rabbit artery preparations (Cambridge et al., 1977a,b). Also, prazosin, unlike yohimbine had little effect on the contractile effect of clonidine at presynaptic α-adrenoceptors in rabbit pulmonary arteries (Cambridge et al., 1978).

In isolated human arteries, prazosin, unlike diazoxide or sodium nitroprusside, had no effect on contractures produced by 5-hydroxytryptamine, angiotensin or $80mmol/L$ potassium chloride (Jauernig and Moulds, 1976; Jauernig et al., 1978). Further, Oates et al. (1976) found that the hypotensive effect of prazosin in doses of 0.1, 1.0 or $10mg/kg$ was completely prevented in rats by pretreatment with pentolinium tartrate or phentolamine, whilst that of diazoxide was not. Prazosin resembled indoramin (an α-adrenoceptor blocking drug) in this regard, and resembled phentolamine in that it caused marked attenuation of the pressor action of noradrenaline, but failed to inhibit angiotensin pressor responses. All three drugs evoked the adrenaline reversal response (Oates et al., 1976; Stokes and Oates, 1977), an effect which had previously been demonstrated for prazosin by Constantine et al. (1973). These findings suggest that the effect of prazosin is one of competitive α-adrenoceptor antagonism rather than direct smooth muscle relaxation.

1.2 Effect on Blood Pressure

Studies in normal and hypertensive rats (Bolli et al., 1975; Constantine et al., 1973; Fernandes et al., 1975), in hypertensive dogs (Constantine et al., 1973; Massingham and Hayden, 1975) and normal dogs (Graham et al., 1976c) have demonstrated the antihypertensive effects of prazosin given orally or intravenously.

Intravenous prazosin,[1] 0.1mg/100g produced a fall in blood pressure which was significant at 30 and 120 minutes in renal and spontaneously hypertensive rats and at 30 minutes in normal rats (Fernandes et al., 1975). In 12 hypertensive dogs, intravenous prazosin 0.1mg/kg and hydrallazine 1mg/kg produced a comparable fall in blood pressure (Massingham and Hayden, 1975). However, acute tolerance to the hypotensive effect of hydrallazine but not the associated tachycardia, was noted within 6 days of daily treatment with oral hydrallazine 2.5mg/kg in conscious hypertensive dogs, but no tolerance occurred in the same time in dogs given oral prazosin 0.625mg/kg (Constantine, 1974). In man, prazosin is 20 to 30 times more potent (weight for weight) than hydrallazine (section 7).

Some tolerance to the antihypertensive effect of oral prazosin 25mg/kg/day in genetically hypertensive rats after 17 days of prazosin administration was noted by Bolli et al. (1975), but this has not been clearly documented during therapeutic use in man (section 7). Wood et al. (1975) reported that 10μg/kg was the threshold dose for a hypotensive effect whether prazosin was injected into the femoral vein or lateral cerebral ventricle. This suggests that the principal antihypertensive effect is not exerted in the central nervous system.

A dose dependent decrease in blood pressure occurred in renal hypertensive rats given prazosin orally in doses of 0.08, 0.32, 1.25 or 5mg/kg and in renal hypertensive dogs given 0.005 to 1.25mg/kg. Following the two highest dosages the hypotensive effect lasted at least 24 hours. Raising the daily dosage about 1mg/kg in hypertensive dogs produced only a slight additional decline in blood pressure. In another group of dogs given 0.075 to 0.625mg/kg daily the maximum hypotensive effect was

---

1   Intravenous prazosin is an experimental dosage form.

achieved on the third day after a dose of 0.31mg/kg body weight (Constantine et al., 1973).

1.3 Effect on Heart Rate

The usual haemodynamic response to a pure vasodilator includes a reflex induced increase in heart rate. Unlike hydrallazine, prazosin does not consistently increase heart rate in animals.

No consistent effect of oral prazosin on the heart rate of hypertensive dogs given single or repeated dosages was recorded by Constantine et al. (1973), but rises of 20 to 25 beats per minute occurred for 2 to 3 minutes after intravenous administration of 0.1 or 0.4mg/kg. Similarly, Massingham and Hayden (1975) found no reflex tachycardia 2 hours after intravenous prazosin 0.1mg/kg or 4 hours after 0.1mg/kg orally in 12 hypertensive dogs, in spite of a fall in blood pressure greater than that obtained with hydrallazine 1mg/kg.

On the other hand, a 33% increase in heart rate by day 3 of a 17 day study in genetically hypertensive rats given prazosin 25mg/kg/day was noted by Bolli et al. (1975). The heart rate remained elevated for the remainder of the study. A significant increase occurred in normal but not in renal hypertensive rats treated by Fernandes et al. (1975); a significant decrease occurred in spontaneously hypertensive rats.

1.4 Effect on Plasma Renin Activity

The effect of prazosin on plasma renin activity (PRA) has varied according to the hypertensive animal model used and possibly may be a function of dosage.

In 12 conscious dogs (Massingham and Hayden, 1975) intravenous prazosin 0.1mg/kg did not produce a significant change in PRA but there was a tendency to increase in a few of the animals. Oral administration of the same dose produced a slight though statistically insignificant increase (3.61 ± 0.28 to 4.11 ± 0.63ng/ml/hr) in conscious dogs. In contrast, a decrease in PRA was reported by Graham et al. (1974, 1976c) in 6 to 7 anaesthetised dogs given prazosin 0.1mg/kg intravenously. A significant fall in PRA by day 4 in genetically hypertensive rats given 25mg/kg daily was recorded by Wood and Lee (1974), but a marked increase in peripheral plasma renin concentration (430 to 470% increase) was reported by Fernandes et al. (1975) in normal Wistar rats given prazosin 0.1mg/100g intravenously. An increase of 79 and 114% at 30 and 120 min respectively occurred in renal hypertensive rats, but in spontaneously hypertensive rats the fall in blood pressure after intravenous prazosin 0.1mg/100g was not associated with a significant change in peripheral plasma renin concentration.

2. Pharmacokinetic Studies in Animals

Studies with ^{14}C-labelled prazosin in dogs (Hess, 1974; Taylor et al., 1976) indicate that the drug is rapidly taken up by the tissues. 30 minutes after a single intravenous injection highest levels of radioactivity were found in the lung (1.23µg/ml). High concentrations of radioactivity were also found in the coronary arteries (1.11µg/g), aorta (0.68µg/g), paw arteries (0.58µg/g) and heart (0.54µg/g) whilst the plasma concentration was 0.174µg/ml at the same time after injection. Brain levels were low (0.028µg/g).

The plasma half-life is reported to be about 1 to 2 hours (Hess, 1974). The hypotensive effect is not related to plasma prazosin levels and persists longer than might be expected from the half-life (Constantine et al., 1973).

Prazosin is extensively metabolised with only about 6% being excreted unchanged in the rat and dog (Taylor et al., 1976). After oral administration of radiolabelled prazosin to dogs and rats, about 4 to 6% and 8 to 10% respectively of the dose is excreted in the urine and the remainder in the faeces; most within 24 hours (Hess, 1974; Taylor et al., 1976). The pattern of excretion after intravenous administration is similar in both the rat and the dog to that after oral dosage. In the rat, about 40% of an intraperitoneal dose was excreted in the bile in 24 hours, whilst in the dog biliary fistula preparation 50% of the oral dose (80% of faecal recovery) was excreted in 72 hours (Taylor et al., 1976). Three of the four metabolites identified are considered to possess about 10 to 25% of the antihypertensive activity of prazosin in dogs (Hess, 1974). The main routes of biotransformation are O-dealkylation and glucuronide formation (Taylor et al., 1976).

3. Human Pharmacology

3.1 Pharmacodynamic Studies

Studies in hypertensive patients have revealed that prazosin has a haemodynamic profile characterised by a significant reduction in total peripheral resistance with no significant increase in cardiac output or heart rate. The pharmacodynamic effects of prazosin have been studied in hypertensive patients after single intravenous[1] or oral doses, and multiple oral doses sufficient to lower blood pressure, given over a short

---

1   Intravenous prazosin is an experimental dosage form and is not commercially available.

period (Safar et al., 1974), or for several weeks (Koshy et al., 1977; Masoni et al., 1974) or months (Ibsen et al., 1977; Lund-Johansen, 1974; 1976).

3.1.1 Single Dose and Short Term Studies

Single intravenous doses administered to hypertensive patients have reduced mean intra-arterial pressure and total peripheral resistance but induced some increase in heart rate (Onesti et al., 1974; Safar et al., 1974; Smith et al., 1974). Changes in cardiac output or cardiac index have been less consistent. An increase in cardiac output from 6.36L/min before prazosin to 6.76L/min after the drug (intravenous dose not stated) was reported by Onesti et al. (1974) in 5 patients, whilst Safar et al. (1974) reported a reduction in cardiac index after intravenous administration of 2mg to 2 patients, and Smith et al. (1975) no change in 2 and a slight increase in the other 2 patients following 0.1mg intravenously. Reduction of cardiac index in the supine position occurred in 5 patients given prazosin in gradually increasing doses up to 20mg over a period of 10 days. However, there was a 4 to 5% increase in cardiac index in the head-up tilt position and during exercise (bicycle ergometer). Following local infusion (Collier et al., 1978), prazosin has a greater dilating effect on veins than on arteries.

3.1.2 Effect of Medium Term Therapy

The haemodynamic effects of 6 to 8 weeks treatment with prazosin 2 to 6mg orally daily were studied by Masoni et al. (1974) in 5 patients with moderate to severe essential hypertension. All patients responded to the drug. Cardiac output increased by an average of 24% and peripheral vascular resistance was significantly reduced by an average of 37%. There was a tendency for venous pressure to be reduced in 4 of 5 patients, while isovolumetric contraction and tension time were reduced in all 5 patients. Koshy et al. (1977), like Masoni et al. (1974) found that prazosin 6 to 15mg daily produced no significant change in cardiac output in 14 outpatients, but plasma volume increased significantly in those whose diastolic blood pressure changed less than 10mm Hg (non-responders). Peripheral resistance was significantly reduced in responders, but not in non-responders. There was no effect on renal function.

3.1.3 Effect of Long Term Therapy

Ten male patients with untreated mild to moderate essential hypertension were studied haemodynamically before and after 11 to 12 months' treatment with prazosin at a dose required to lower blood pressure (3 to 7.5mg daily). The haemodynamic changes are summarised in table II. The most impressive finding was a significant reduction in blood pressure and total peripheral resistance at rest, sitting and during exercise. The change in cardiac index at rest for the group as a whole was not significant and neither was the change in heart rate at rest or during exercise or in stroke in-

Table II. Changes in haemodynamic variables in patients showing an adequate hypotensive response during long term oral therapy of hypertension with prazosin (after Lund-Johansen, 1974)

Variable	% Change[1] at rest (supine)	Exercise		
		300kpm/ min	600kpm/ min	900kpm/ min
Systolic pressure (mm Hg)	↓(9)[2]	↓(10.5%)	↓(10%)	↓(8.5%)
Diastolic pressure (mm Hg)	↓(9.5)	↓(11%)	↓(8.5%)	↓(8.5%)
Total peripheral resistance index (dyn/sec/cm^{-5}m^2	↓(15)	↓(21%)	↓(22%)	↓(23%)
Cardiac index (L/min/m^2)	↑(8)	↑(15%)	↑(12%)	↑(12.5%)
Stroke index (ml/stroke/m^2)	↑(8)	↑(11%)	↑(8%)	↑(10.5%)
Heart rate (beats/min)	↔	↑(4%)	↑(4%)	↑(2.5%)

1   ↓ = decrease; ↑ = increase; ↔ no change.

2   Figure in parenthesis indicates percentage change.

dex at rest (Lund-Johansen, 1974). In another group of similar patients prazosin was used in combination with tolamolol for 7 to 12 months. The fall in blood pressure at rest was due to a fall in cardiac index and peripheral resistance. During exercise the cardiac index was not significantly lowered, but there was a significant fall in peripheral resistance (Lund-Johansen, 1977).

Ibsen et al. (1977) reported a significant increase in plasma volume and extracellular volume in 8 hypertensives in whom prazosin (mean dose 11mg daily) was added to propranolol therapy for a period of 3 to 4 months. These changes were reversed by the addition of hydrochlorothiazide. There was no significant change in renal function.

3.2 Effect on Renal Function

Single doses of prazosin given orally or intravenously[1] (Maxwell, 1974) and therapeutic doses administered for several weeks (Masoni et al., 1974; Koshy et al., 1977) or months (Ibsen et al., 1977) to small groups of hypertensive patients, have produced no demonstrable deterioration in renal function.

1   Intravenous prazosin is an experimental dosage form and is not commercially available.

In the 5 patients with moderate to severe hypertension treated by Masoni et al. (1974) for 6 to 8 weeks, blood urea nitrogen was practically unchanged, but showed a slight decrease in 4 patients. Creatinine clearance, glomerular filtration rate and renal plasma volume all increased slightly, but the extent to which blood pressure had been controlled before the study is not known.

No impairment of renal fluid and electrolyte metabolism was observed by Maxwell (1974) in 4 patients with essential hypertension given a single intravenous dose in doses ranging from 0.06 to 13mg, although in this study the fall in blood pressure was only small and may not indicate the effect of the drug on renal function following a substantial fall in blood pressure.

The lack of adverse effect of prazosin on renal function in these studies has been confirmed in therapeutic trials involving hypertensive patients with impaired renal function (section 5.6).

3.3 Effect on Plasma Renin Activity

Plasma renin activity (PRA) has consistently been reduced in hypertensive patients treated with therapeutic doses of prazosin alone for at least 4 weeks (Feng et al., 1975; Hayes et al., 1976b).

A decrease of 62 % in the mean PRA was recorded by Hayes et al. (1976b, 1977) in 9 hypertensive patients treated for a mean period of 28 days at a mean dose of 7.9mg. There was no correlation between the reduction in PRA and the hypotensive response. A 40 % mean fall in PRA in 8 patients treated with prazosin 2 to 9mg daily was reported by Feng et al. (1975). The increase in PRA normally expected with administration of a thiazide diuretic is reduced by concomitant prazosin. Combined administration of 0.5g chlorothiazide and prazosin in 8 patients improved control of blood pressure and resulted in a mean increase of only 7 % in PRA, which is lower than expected with the thiazide alone, (Feng et al., 1975). The addition of prazosin in patients treated with polythiazide resulted in a reduction in PRA (Steele and Lowenstein, 1976). The effect of prazosin may be influenced by the initial level of PRA, which was high (13.1 ± 7.7) in the study of Hayes et al. (1976b) and much lower (2.31 ± 1.74) in the study of Feng et al. (1975).

4. Pharmacokinetic Studies in Man

4.1 Absorption

Studies of the pharmacokinetics of prazosin in man are few. Available data indicate that prazosin is readily absorbed after oral administration but that there is considerable variation between individual subjects in the peak serum concentration and the time required to attain it, although the pattern of absorption is consistent within each individual. Also the effect of food on serum concentrations varies between individuals. Serum levels are increased by food in some subjects and reduced in others. It is highly protein bound and has a large volume of distribution.

Fasting mean peak serum concentrations of 23 ± 10.5ng/ml were reported by Verbesselt et al. (1976) in 18 subjects 1 to 2 hours after a single oral dose of prazosin 2mg (tablet), whilst Wood et al. (1976) recorded the same mean level (23 ± 10.5ng/ml) 2 to 3 hours after a single 5mg oral dose (tablet). Serum levels at other dosage levels were not studied in either study. In another group of 24 healthy volunteers, mean peak serum levels of 36 ± 17.3ng/ml were attained at about 2 hours (with a range of 6.2 to 78.4ng/ml at 1 to 4 hours) following a single 5mg oral dose given as one capsule (Hobbs and Twomey, 1977). Initial peak plasma levels are said to be lower following oral administration as capsules than as tablets (Norris, 1977, personal communication).

In a repeated dose study in 4 hypertensive volunteers, peak plasma levels of 14.9 ± 3.5ng/ml were attained on day 1 after a 2mg oral dose, whereas peak concentrations averaged 26.8 ± ng/ml on day 4 following 2mg 3 times daily on days 2 and 3 and 2mg on day 4 (Graham et al., 1976b). Collins and Pek (1975). Collins and Pek (1975) reported that peak serum levels (unstated value) of prazosin in 5 hypertensive patients were attained 1.5 to 5h (mean 3.6h) after a single 2 to 5mg oral dose.

Although food did not significantly alter the mean peak serum concentration of prazosin or the time at which it was attained, both of these variables differed considerably between individuals (Verbesselt et al., 1976). In 9 subjects the serum levels were higher when prazosin was given after food (either breakfast or a substantial lunch) than after fasting, whilst in 7 the serum levels were reduced in the presence of food.

4.2 Distribution

Prazosin is bound to human plasma proteins to the extent of 97 % (Hobbs and Twomey, 1977), and has an apparent volume of distribution of approximately 75 litres (Hobbs and Twomey, 1977) or 118 litres (Wood, 1974).

4.3 Elimination

Preliminary metabolic studies with unlabelled prazosin (Taylor et al., 1976) indicate a pattern of hepatic metabolic degradation similar to that in dogs (section 2). Mean liver extraction was estimated to be 29.9 % and the mean hepatic clearance 448ml/min (Collins and Pek, 1975).

Plasma concentration declines according to first order kinetics with a mean half-life of about 2.5 to 5 hours (Collins and Pek, 1975; Hobbs and Twomey, 1977; Lowenthal et al., 1978; Simpson et al., 1977; Wood, 1974; Wood et al., 1976) and a range in half-life of 1.77 to 4.55 (Hobbs and Twomey, 1977). Following multiple doses, a significant shortening of half-life with 1 and 2mg doses but not with 5mg, was noted by Lowenthal et al. (1978) when compared with single doses in the same patients. Simpson et al. (1977) observed that the half-life in patients receiving maintenance therapy may be longer than in normal volunteers.

4.4 Plasma Concentration and Clinical Effects

The blood pressure lowering effect of prazosin is said not to be closely related to the plasma concentration of the drug (Wood, 1974) and in another study designed to investigate the 'first dose' reaction (section 8.1), the peak plasma concentration coincided with the maximal hypotensive response on day 1 but preceded the maximal response on day 4; the first dose hypotensive response subsiding by day 4 despite the presence of much higher plasma concentrations (Graham et al., 1976b). The antihypertensive effect of prazosin persists for longer (about 10 hours) than expected from the short plasma half-life (Wood, 1974); a finding common to other antihypertensive drugs such as methyldopa and propranolol.

4.5 Influence of Disease on Kinetics

Markedly elevated plasma levels of prazosin and prolonged disappearance of the drug from the plasma have been reported in 2 hypertensive patients with renal impairment, one of whom was also receiving propranolol (Collins and Pek, 1975; Graham et al., 1976b). This suggests a reduced hepatic extraction of prazosin in patients with chronic renal impairment as a consequence of the disease, and in one of the cases, perhaps also to the contribution of propranolol in decreasing hepatic blood flow. Reduced hepatic extraction in patients with chronic renal failure has also been reported for propranolol itself (Bianchetti et al., 1976). Bioavailability of propranolol was also increased in chronic renal failure patients not on dialysis and indicates that the first-pass hepatic metabolism of orally administered propranolol is considerably reduced in patients with renal failure. Collins and Pek (1975) have suggested that prazosin is also subject to significant first-pass metabolism. This aspect requires further investigation. Whatever the mechanism for the higher and more prolonged plasma levels in chronic renal failure, smaller than usual doses of prazosin should be given, especially initially (see also section 6.2).

Table III. Results and design of therapeutic trials comparing prazosin and placebo in patients with hypertension

Author	No. pats.	Dose (daily)	Design[1]	Duration[2]	Results[3]
Bolli et al. (1976)	12	1.5-38mg (1.5 to 10mg in 11 patients)	d-b within patient	6 weeks	Supine; 17/8 lower with prazosin Standing; 24/14 lower with prazosin
Mroczek and Finnerty (1974)	39	16.5mg av (20mg in 11/21 on prazosin)	d-b between patient	12 weeks	Supine; 18/9 lower with prazosin Standing; 19/12 lower with prazosin
Schnaper and Oberman (1975)	22	19.2mg av (range 15 to 20mg)	d-b between patient	12 weeks	Supine; 10/5 lower with prazosin Standing; 14/8 lower with prazosin

1 d-b = double blind; within patient = cross-over design.
2 Duration on each medication.
3 Blood pressure measurements expressed in mm Hg and compared with baseline readings.

5. Therapeutic Trials

Therapeutic trials conducted throughout the world have demonstrated the efficacy of prazosin in reducing all grades of hypertension either when used alone in cases of mild to moderate severity or in combination with a diuretic and/or other antihypertensive drugs in moderate to severe cases.

Prazosin has been shown to be as satisfactory as α-methyldopa in controlling blood pressure when the dosage of both drugs was increased until either the blood pressure was controlled or an arbitary maximum dose was reached (section 5.2).

The efficacy of prazosin is increased by the addition of the thiazide diuretic, polythiazide (section 5.3). Although there are no suitably designed studies comparing the efficacy of prazosin alone with prazosin plus other thiazide diuretics, there is no reason to believe that they are less suitable than polythiazide.

The addition of prazosin to other antihypertensive drugs which have failed to control the blood pressure has often resulted in satisfactory control without any increase in side effects (section 5.4).

5.1 Prazosin Compared with Placebo

In between-patient (Mroczek and Finnerty 1974; Schnaper and Oberman, 1975) and within-patient (Bolli et al., 1976) comparisons of prazosin and placebo the antihypertensive response to the active drug has been consistently better than that to placebo (table III).

In nearly all studies the dose of prazosin has been increased until the diastolic pressure was reduced to 90mm Hg or lower or until a chosen maximum dose (usually 20mg daily) was reached or side effects intervened. All but 3 of the patients in the study of Bolli et al. (1976) were receiving one or more antihypertensive drugs before the trial in addition to prazosin. Apart from prazosin, antihypertensive therapy was kept constant throughout the 6 weeks on placebo or prazosin. The total number of tablets taken during the trial was the same as before it. The hypotensive effect of prazosin as compared with placebo was not related to the severity of hypertension or to the nature or amount of concomitant antihypertensive therapy. Although in this study there was no relation between hypotensive effect and dose of prazosin, Pitts (1975) reported an increased percentage response rate with an increase in dosage.

A delay of 6 or 8 weeks before there was a demonstrable effect of prazosin on diastolic pressure was noted by Mroczek and Finnerty (1974) in their black American patients, and a delayed onset of maximal effect of several weeks was mentioned by Schnaper and Obermann (1975) and by Bolzano (1974), particularly in patients with a long history of hypertension and who had not received effective therapy. This delay before the full effects of prazosin became apparent has also been observed by other workers. In the study of Schnaper and Oberman (1975) normalisation of supine diastolic pressure (< 90mm Hg) was achieved in 5 of 10 patients treated with prazosin and in 1 of 12 given placebo. A reduction of diastolic pressure to below 100mm Hg was achieved in 50 % of the 10 prazosin patients and in 8.3 % of the 12 given placebo.

5.2 Prazosin Compared with α-Methyldopa

Several studies conducted in different parts of the world in patients with largely mild (diastolic 90 to 99mm Hg) to moderate (diastolic 100 to 114mm Hg) essential hypertension have compared the antihypertensive effects of prazosin with those of α-methyldopa (table IV). In only five of these studies has the dosage of each drug been titrated to achieve optimum control of blood pressure (Bloom et al., 1975; Bradley et al., 1977; Fernandes et al., 1975; Mroczek and Finnerty, 1974; Smith et al., 1975), other studies having used fixed doses of each drug. In the two within-patient studies which have titrated the dosage (Bloom et al., 1975; Smith et al., 1975) there has been little to choose between the two drugs with respect to either antihypertensive efficacy or incidence of troublesome side effects.

Table IV. Results and design of therapeutic trials comparing prazosin with α-methyldopa in patients with mostly mild to moderate essential hypertension

Author	No. pats.	Daily dosage (mg)	Study design¹	Duration²	Results (satisfactory control)	
					Prazosin	α-Methyldopa
Amery et al. (1974)	23	Pr 3 αM 750	d-b within patient	6 weeks	Reduction in BP not significant	Reduction in BP statistically significant
Bradley et al. (1977)	45	Pr 3-20 (mean 8.5) αM 750-3,000 (mean 1,183)	d-b; s-b patient	14 weeks	Diastolic pressure $<$ 100mm Hg in 75% of 22	Diastolic pressure $<$ 100mm Hg in 47.4% of 23
Bloom et al. (1975)	30	Pr 9.5 ± 0.8 (mean) αM 1,325 ± 97 mean	d-b within patient	10 weeks	Reduction to $<$ 100mm Hg diastolic in 16/25	Reduction to $<$ 100mm Hg diastolic in 17/27
Fernandes et al. (1975)	53	Pr $<$ 20 αM $<$ 2,000	d-b between patient	12 weeks	Average mean arterial pressure reduced 12%	Average mean arterial pressure reduced 16%
Guevara-Viales (1976)	40	Pr 5-15 αM 750 to 1,500	d-b between patient	8 months	'Normal' in 20/20	'Normal' in 19/20
Mroczek and Finnerty (1974)	42	Pr 16.5 (av) αM 1,190 (av)	d-b between patient	12 weeks	Reduction to $<$ 90mm Hg diastolic in 7/21; to $<$ 100 mm Hg in 14/21	Reduction to $<$ 90mm Hg diastolic in 10/21; to $<$ 100mm Hg in 15/21

Study	N	Dose	Design	Duration[2]	Result (Prazosin)	Result (αMethyldopa)
Piza Lopez and Gutierrez Fuster (1975)	60	Pr 3-6 αM 750-1,500	d-b between patient	6 months	Diastolic pressure <90mm Hg in 25 (78%) of 32	Diastolic pressure <90mm Hg in 20 (71%) of 28
Schnaper and Oberman (1975)	39	Pr 3 αM 750	d-b between patient	6 weeks	Reduction to <90mm Hg diastolic in 8/20; to <100 mm Hg in 15/20	Reduction to <90mm Hg diastolic in 5/19; to <100mm Hg in 11/19
Stokes and Weber (1974)	15	Pr 3 to 7.5 αM 750	d-b within patient	5.2 to 9.6 weeks	Mean arterial pressure reduced to <110mm Hg or to >15mm Hg below control in 9/15	Mean arterial pressure reduced to <110mm Hg or to >15mm Hg below control in 9/15
Smith et al. (1975)	33	Pr 3 to 20 αM 750 to 2,000	d-b within patient	12 weeks	Mean arterial pressure reduced by 12%	Mean arterial pressure reduced by 16%
Venables and Duff (1974)	24	Pr 6 αM 750	s-b within patient	>4 weeks	Satisfactory control (not defined) in 11/17	Satisfactory control (not defined) in 8/17
Vryens and Adrianensen (1974)	20[3]	Pr 3 αM 750	d-b within patient	6 weeks	Reduction to <90mm Hg in 13/20	Reduction to 90mm Hg in 9/20

1 Double blind = d-b; single-blind = s-b
2 Duration of therapy with each drug
3 Combined patients from 2 studies each with 10 patients

Reduction of mean standing diastolic pressure to 100mm Hg or below, or to at least 41mm Hg below the control, was reported by Bloom et al. (1975) in 16 of 25 patients whilst receiving prazosin and in 17 of 27 during therapy with α-methyldopa. Prazosin failed to influence blood pressure in two patients whilst there were no complete failures with methyldopa. A mean arterial pressure of 137mm Hg in 33 patients with essential hypertension treated by Smith et al. (1975), was reduced to 115 by α-methyldopa and to 121mm Hg by prazosin in the supine position and to 109 and 120mm Hg respectively in the standing position.

In a between-patient study conducted in black Americans by Mroczek and Finnerty (1974) in 42 patients with mild to moderate essential hypertension, reduction of supine diastolic blood pressure to less than 90mm Hg was achieved in 7 (33%) treated with prazosin and in 10 (48%) treated with α-methyldopa. Resistance to the antihypertensive effects of prazosin in daily dosages of up to 6mg was noted in Nigerian patients by Falase et al. (1976) but not by Oviasu et al. (1976) [section 5.3]. In a multicentre study conducted in America (race not stated), Bradley et al. (1977) reported that supine diastolic blood pressure was reduced to below 100mm Hg in 75% of 22 patients treated with prazosin and in 43% of 23 patients treated with α-methyldopa.

Studies employing fixed doses of prazosin and α-methyldopa have attempted to establish a ratio of potency for the two drugs, but not surprisingly, in view of the differences between the drugs in their dosage range and mechanism of action, findings have varied. The method of increasing the dosage of the drug until response is adequate, the maximum dosage is reached or until side effects intervene is likely to reveal more useful information regarding the relative antihypertensive effectiveness of the drugs, than the use of fixed dosages.

Whereas Amery et al. (1974) found 750mg daily of α-methyldopa to be more effective in lowering blood pressure in 23 patients with grade I or II (WHO criteria) than 3mg daily of prazosin (these data also reported by Verhiest et al., 1974), Schnaper and Oberman (1975), who used the same fixed dosages, reported a reduction of supine diastolic pressure to below 90mm Hg in 43% of the 20 patients treated with prazosin and in 37.5% of the 19 who received α-methyldopa. In the study of Verhiest et al. (1974) and Amery et al. (1974), the dosage of prazosin may have been too low, as 7.5mg daily produced a significant fall in blood pressure in a group of 15 of the same patients treated after completion of the double-blind trial. These workers found a correlation between the fall in blood pressure during each period which suggested that the patients whose systolic pressure decreased most with α-methyldopa also experienced greater decreases with prazosin, and vice versa. Unlike Verhiest et al. (1974), Vryens and Adriasensen (1974) found that 3mg daily of prazosin tended to be more effective than α-methyldopa 750mg daily in 20 patients with mild to moderate essential hypertension. Normalisation of blood pressure (< 90mm Hg) was achieved in 13 of 20 patients during prazosin therapy and in 9 of 20 during α-methyldopa.

In contrast, Stokes and Weber (1974) found that response to prazosin, α-methyldopa and propranolol varied between the 12 individuals studied. Two patients failed to respond to any of the drugs and three who did not respond to prazosin responded to the other two drugs. Only 5 patients responded to all three drugs and in 2 of these α-methyldopa had to be withdrawn because of side effects. These investigators found that the antihypertensive effect of prazosin 3 to 7.5mg daily was comparable with that of 750mg daily of α-methyldopa.

Venables and Duff (1974), in a single-blind within-patient study in 17 patients (8 moderate; 9 severe), reported control of blood pressure to be 'satisfactory' (not defined) in 11 (64.7%) during prazosin and in 8 (47%) whilst receiving α-methyldopa. Although the dose of α-methyldopa could be increased to 2g daily, comparison of efficacy was made on the assumption that 6mg daily of prazosin is equivalent to 750mg α-methyldopa.

Thus, on the basis of present evidence it appears that the antihypertensive effectiveness of prazosin is comparable with that of α-methyldopa when the dosage of both drugs is adjusted to achieve optimum control of blood pressure. In the studies reported so far, the overall incidence of side effects and the proportion necessitating withdrawal of therapy have been similar with both drugs (section 8.5).

5.3 Prazosin plus a Thiazide Diuretic Compared with Prazosin Alone

The combined use of a thiazide diuretic with prazosin results in an increased antihypertensive effect over and above that obtained with either drug alone. In most studies conducted so far, the thiazide has been added to the maximum dose of prazosin in patients who have not shown an adequate response to prazosin alone (table V), but there is no clear evidence that this is preferable to giving the thiazide first and then adding prazosin (see also section 7). While in practically all studies, polythiazide has been the thiazide employed, other thiazides can of course be used equally as well.

In the only study designed to specifically compare the effects of prazosin plus a thiazide with those of both drugs alone in the same patients (Cohen, 1970), the combination of polythiazide plus prazosin was more effective than either drug alone at similar dosages (fig. 2). As might be expected, the effect of the combination was most evident in patients with more severe hypertension, although in this study normalisation of the blood pressure was achieved in an increased proportion of patients with all levels of hypertension when given combined therapy. The difference in response between the combination and prazosin alone was less marked in the study of Bradley (1975), but this study involved few patients with severe hypertension.

The extent to which the final dosage of prazosin can be reduced when a thiazide is added is not clear from present data, but in the study of Rougier et al. (1974) results suggested that prazosin 6mg daily plus 1 to 3mg daily of polythiazide was at least as

Table V. Results and design of therapeutic trials in hypertensive patients treated with prazosin and polythiazide

Author	Population[1]	Daily dosage	Duration	Results and comments
Bradley (1975)	50 mild 28 mod 19 severe 3	Prazosin: <20mg Polythiazide: 2 to 4mg	42 months	Supine diastolic <90mm Hg: in 8/16 who completed 42 months on prazosin alone in 11/13 who completed 42 months on prazosin + polythiazide
Cohen (1970)	38 mild 12 mod 14 severe 10 gross 2	Prazosin: 8 to 40mg Polythiazide: 2mg	2 to 4 weeks on any one regimen	Supine diastolic <90mm Hg: in 9/38 during prazosin alone in 8/38 during polythiazide alone in 33/38 during prazosin + polythiazide
de la Paz et al. (1975)	29 mild 7 mod 16 severe 6	Prazosin: <20mg Polythiazide (NS)[2] (30.4 mean)	10 to 60 weeks (30.4 mean)	Marked response, 30/15mm Hg fall: in 5/9 who failed to respond adequately to up to 20mg prazosin alone
de la Paz et al. (1976)	114 mild 24 mod 68 severe 22	Prazosin <20mg Polythiazide	6 to 60 weeks (7.5 months mean)	Blood pressure reduced by combined treatment to 140/90mm Hg or below in 34 of 56 patients who failed to respond to prazosin alone
Falase et al. (1976)	15 mild 9[3] mod 3 severe 3	Prazosin: 6 to 15mg Polythiazide: 3mg	<24 weeks	Further reduction in diastolic blood pressure of 5 to 35mm Hg in 11/14 in whom polythiazide added
Fernandes et al. (1975)	48	Prazosin: <20mg Polythiazide: 2mg	3 to 8 months	Supine diastolic blood pressure reduced in 28/48 patients unresponsive to 20mg prazosin from average of 109 to 92mm Hg
Mabadeje (1978)	40 mild 6 mod 25 severe 9	Prazosin: <30mg[5] Polythiazide: 2mg	6 months	Blood pressure reduced to <140/90mm Hg in 6 with moderate and 2 with severe hypertension who had shown a lesser response to prazosin alone

Study	No. of patients	Dosage	Duration	Results
Maher (1975)	20 mild 8[4] mod 7 severe 5	Prazosin: <20mg Polythiazide: <4mg	3 to 10 months	A further reduction in blood pressure in 6 of 11 patients who failed to respond to prazosin alone, many of whom had been treated with three or more antihypertensive agents before the trial
Oviasu and Idahosa (1976)	14	Prazosin 4 to 6mg Hydrochlorothiazide 50mg	24 to 30 weeks	Blood pressure (supine) reduced by mean value of 44/24.5mm Hg by prazosin plus hydrochlorothiazide and by 12.5/11.4mm Hg by prazosin alone
Rab and Farooqui (1975)	37 mild 2 mod 20 severe 7 gross 8	Prazosin: 4 to 18mg Polythiazide: 1 to 2mg	6 months	Supine blood pressure reduced to 130/90: in 11/37 during prazosin in 14/37 during prazosin plus polythiazide
Rougier et al. (1974)	118 mild 22 mod 58 severe 38	Prazosin: <15mg Polythiazide: 1 to 3mg	16 weeks	Blood pressure reduced to >90 to <100mm Hg in 25/34 treated with 6mg prazosin + polythiazide and in 10/24 treated with 15mg prazosin alone. All 58 had failed to respond to prazosin 6mg alone

1 Mild hypertension = diastolic of 90-99mm Hg; moderate hypertension = diastolic of 100-114mm Hg; severe hypertension = diastolic of 115-129mm Hg; gross hypertension = diastolic of 130 and over mm Hg.
2 NS = not stated.
3 Mild hypertension = diastolic 90-105mm Hg; moderate hypertension = diastolic of 106-120mm Hg; severe hypertension = 120 and over mm Hg.
4 Mild hypertension 90-104mm Hg.
5 One patient received 60mg prazosin.

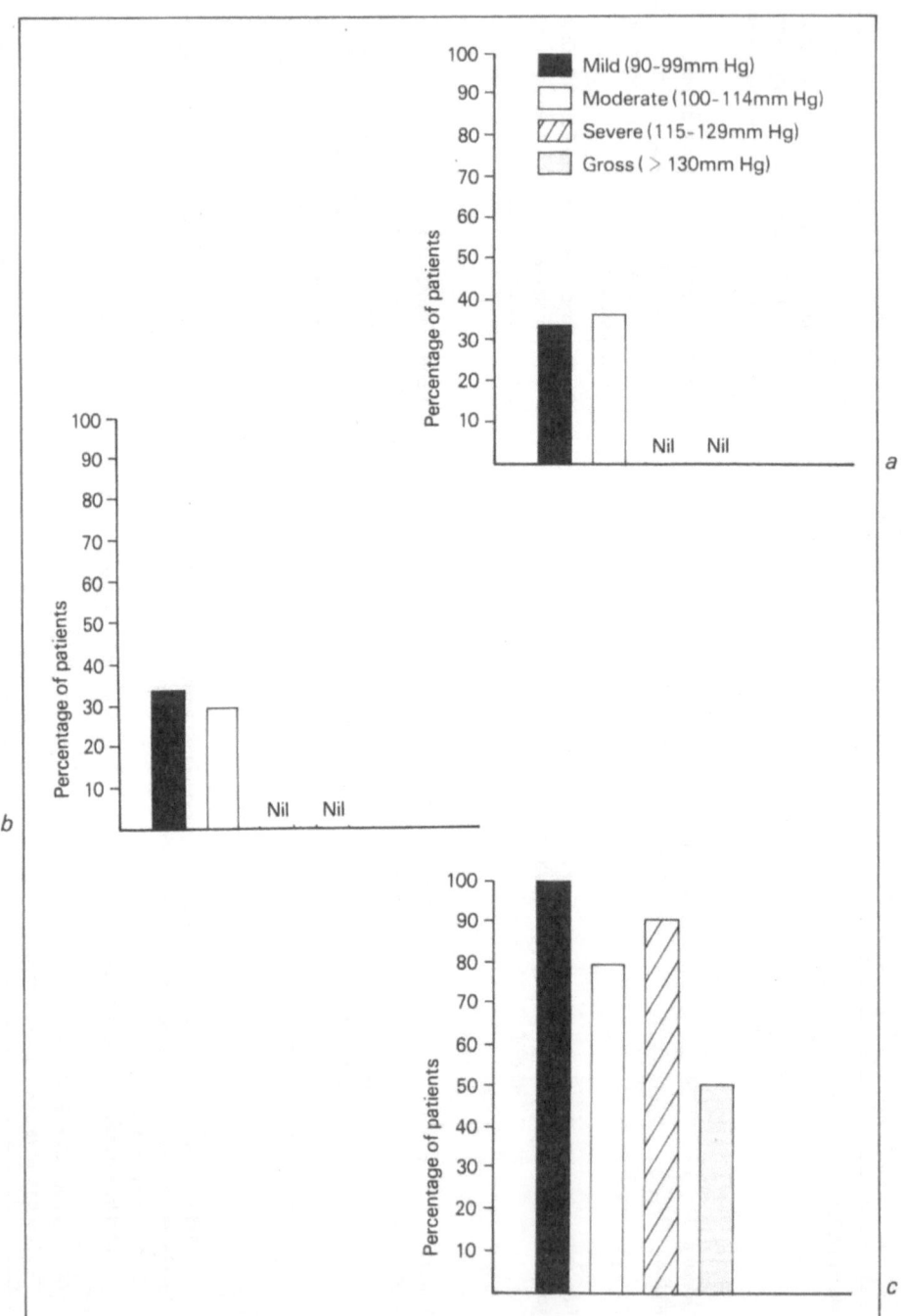

effective in lowering blood pressure as prazosin 15mg alone (table V). 58 patients in whom control of blood pressure was less than satisfactory on prazosin 6mg daily, were given either prazosin 6mg plus 1 to 3mg polythiazide daily or prazosin 15mg daily. Supine diastolic blood pressure was reduced to 90mm Hg or below in 4 (12%) of 34 given prazosin plus polythiazide and in 1 (4%) of 24 given prazosin 15mg alone. A supine diastolic blood pressure of 100mm Hg or below was achieved in 21 (74%) of 34 given prazosin 6mg plus polythiazide and in 10 (42%) of 24 given prazosin 15mg daily alone. Side effects were reported in 46 instances among 84 patients who received prazosin 6 to 15mg daily and in 12 instances in the 34 patients who received the prazosin-polythiazide combination.

A difficult test of the effectiveness of prazosin was provided in the study of Maher (1975). 16 of the 20 patients had previously been treated for their hypertension with other drugs and most had required treatment with a combination of antihypertensive agents. Prazosin was initially given in a dose of up to 15mg daily and those who failed to respond were given prazosin plus a thiazide (polythiazide) or placebo in addition to their prazosin. Prazosin alone was as effective as the combination in patients with mild disease (mean baseline blood pressure 161/106mm Hg) but a further average reduction of 18/8mm Hg was achieved by the addition of polythiazide in 11 patients with more severe disease (mean baseline blood pressure 187/111mm Hg). 2 patients failed to respond to maximum doses of the combined drugs (prazosin 20mg; polythiazide 4mg), but 3 patients who had previously required 3 or 4 drugs including guanethidine, responded as well or better to prazosin plus polythiazide. Falase et al. (1976), found that prazosin 6mg daily failed to produce a statistically significant fall in supine or erect blood pressure in Nigerian patients, but in other studies, Oviasu and Idahosa (1976), Mabadeje (1978) and Salim et al. (1977) reported a satisfactory response in patients from Nigeria and Tanzania. In one study (Oviasu and Idahosa, 1976), prazosin 15mg daily reduced blood pressure significantly only in the erect position, whereas prazosin 6mg and 15mg plus a thiazide (polythiazide 3mg) daily reduced supine blood pressure significantly. Mabadeje (1978) reported that sitting blood pressure was reduced by prazosin alone to 140/90mm Hg or less in all 9 with mild hypertension, in 19 (76%) with moderate and 33% with severe disease. The addition of polythiazide 2mg daily increased the response rate to 100% in those with moderate hypertension and to 55% in severe hypertension.

Prazosin adds to the antihypertensive response induced by initial thiazide diuretic therapy and some investigators have commenced therapy in this way. In 20 patients

---

Fig. 2. Percentage of patients with mild, moderate, severe or gross hypertension (defined in mm Hg diastolic) whose supine blood pressure was reduced to 150/90mm Hg or below during 4 week's therapy with prazosin (A), 2 week's therapy with polythiazide (B) or 4 week's therapy with prazosin plus polythiazide (C) [after Cohen, 1970].

with essential hypertension of varying severity (gross, 8; severe, 4; moderate, 6 and mild, 2) a reduction of 25.3/10.6mm Hg was achieved with a thiazide alone (polythiazide 4mg daily) compared with the placebo period (Oh et al., 1974). A further reduction of 8/8.1mm Hg was achieved by the addition of prazosin 6mg daily and of 19.5/14.5 by the addition of 20mg daily. Diastolic blood pressure was reduced to 90mm Hg or below in 4 of 12 whose hypertension was gross[2] or severe and in 6 of 8 with moderate to mild disease.

In a multicentre trial in 114 hypertensive patients, de la Paz et al. (1976) reported that the addition of a thiazide (polythiazide) to prazosin produced a satisfactory response (< 140/90mm Hg) in 24 of 56 patients unresponsive to prazosin alone. In a study in 25 hypertensives mostly with moderate disease, Reyes (1974) also reported the reduction of blood pressure to 140/90mm Hg or below in 15 patients given polythiazide plus prazosin who had failed to respond adequately to 20mg daily prazosin alone.

Pitkajarvi et al. (1977) began treatment of hypertension in 43 newly diagnosed male patients with a thiazide and added prazosin (6 to 15mg) or the β-adrenoceptor blocking drug tolamolol (300 to 600mg) or both of these drugs in those whose diastolic pressure remained above 100mm Hg. Polythiazide (1mg daily) plus prazosin or tolamolol controlled hypertension in 31 of the 38 patients who failed to respond to polythiazide alone. Hypertension was more severe in the 7 patients who required the triple drug regimen but all responded. Results with polythiazide plus prazosin were comparable with those of the polythiazide-tolamolol combination. Similar findings were reported by Kim (1976) in 30 patients with moderate to severe hypertension which had failed to respond to previous antihypertensive therapy. 6 patients responded to prazosin 6mg daily, 17 to prazosin 6 to 15mg plus a thiazide (polythiazide 3mg daily) and the remaining 7 to a combination of prazosin, polythiazide and the β-blocker tolamolol. In this study, polythiazide was added after only 1 week's treatment with a fixed dose of 6mg daily of prazosin, and a greater proportion of the patients may have responded to prazosin alone had it been continued for a longer period (section 5.1).

Although in the studies of Kim (1976) and Pitkajarvi et al. (1977), there was a tendency for patients with severely elevated blood pressure to require combined treatment with prazosin plus a thiazide and/or a β-blocker, no such tendency was evident in the study of Seedat et al. (1977). These investigators found that prazosin alone in doses of up to 20mg daily (mean 5.7mg twice daily) reduced diastolic blood pressure by 20mm Hg or more or to 110mm Hg or less in 22 of 25 patients. 24 of these patients had severe (diastolic pressure 115 to 129mm Hg) or gross (> 130mm Hg) hypertension. All 20 patients in another group (3 moderate; 8 severe; 9 gross) treated

---

2   Definition of 'gross' hypertension not stated but blood pressure was elevated to a greater extent than those in the 'severe' group.

with prazosin (mean 4.4mg twice daily) plus the thiazide diuretic cyclopenthiazide 0.5mg daily were considered to have responded satisfactorily. The mean blood pressure was 178/127mm Hg before therapy and 140/93mm Hg after prazosin alone, and 174/124mm Hg and 137/95mm Hg before and after treatment with prazosin and cyclopenthiazide.

Further studies comparing prazosin alone with thiazide-prazosin regimens using reduced doses of prazosin, are needed to determine whether there is any advantage in adding the thiazide before the maximum dosage of prazosin is reached, or whether it is more useful to commence therapy with a thiazide and then add prazosin (see also section 7).

5.4 Prazosin Compared with Hydrallazine

Studies comparing prazosin and hydrallazine in hypertensive patients also receiving other antihypertensive agents indicated that prazosin 1mg had an effect about the same as 20mg to 30mg hydrallazine (Hua et al., 1977a,b; Kincaid-Smith et al., 1977; Rasmussen and Jensen 1976; 1977). Side effects necessitating withdrawal of the drug occurred more frequently with hydrallazine than with prazosin (Kincaid-Smith et al., 1977).

In a 12-week study involving 8 patients whose blood pressure was not adequately controlled by propranolol and chlorothiazide, prazosin (1mg capsules) and hydrallazine (25mg capsules) were given in doses sufficient to lower diastolic blood pressure to below 95mm Hg. Blood pressure fell by 14.7/15.8mm Hg (supine) and 24.2/13.1mm Hg (standing) during prazosin, and by 20.7/16.2mm Hg (supine) and 23.8/16.2mm Hg (standing) during hydrallazine treatment. In a 6-week study, 8 of 24 patients were withdrawn because of side effects. Seven were unable to tolerate side effects whilst on hydrallazine (severe headache, palpitations, flushing, burning sensation in the eyes, nausea and vomiting) but side effects (marked dizziness) necessitated cessation of prazosin in only one patient (Hua et al., 1977a; Hua, 1977, personal communication; Kincaid-Smith, 1975; Kincaid-Smith et al., 1977). Prazosin in a mean dose of 5.46mg had an antihypertensive effect similar to that of hydrallazine in a mean dose of 163mg in 15 outpatients also receiving propranolol. Mean duration of prazosin treatment was 7 months (Rasmussen and Jensen, 1976; 1977).

5.5 Prazosin in Combination with other Antihypertensive Drugs

Several studies have shown prazosin to be particularly useful when added to existing antihypertensive therapy in patients in whom control of blood pressure was inadequate or side effects were preventing further dose increments. Prazosin has been used in conjunction with β-adrenoceptor blocking agents, diuretics, clonidine, α-methyldopa or hydrallazine when these drugs were given alone or in various combinations.

As most patients treated with combinations of antihypertensive drugs have severe hypertension, the use of placebo is often not desirable and consequently most studies in these patients have not been placebo controlled.

In a within-patient controlled trial, Marshall et al. (1977) compared the effects of adding bendrofluazide (5 to 10mg daily) or prazosin (6 to 15mg daily), or both drugs to a β-adrenoceptor blocking drug in 20 patients who had an inadequate fall in blood pressure after at least 2 months therapy with β-blockade alone. An additional fall in supine blood pressure of 10 to 11 % resulted from the addition of bendrofluazide and of 13 % when prazosin was added. There was no significant difference between the effect of 5 and 10mg of bendrofluazide a day and the fall in blood pressure after 2 weeks was not significantly different from that at 8 weeks. On the other hand, increasing the daily dose of prazosin from 6 to 15mg resulted in a further significant decrease in blood pressure compared with that achieved by adding either drug alone. However, the fall achieved by giving both prazosin and bendrofluazide together was not significantly different from that expected if the falls produced by the two drugs individually were added.

Bolli and Simpson (1975) verified the efficacy of prazosin by reducing its dosage after the optimum dose had been reached. Prazosin therapy resulted in a considerable reduction in blood pressure in nearly all patients. 6 of the 24 patients received prazosin alone whilst the others had previously been treated with a diuretic alone (3), a β-adrenoceptor blocking drug alone or with a diuretic (9), or with a diuretic plus one or more other antihypertensive agents (6). There was a postural fall in blood pressure before prazosin was started in all groups of patients but the addition of prazosin to the treatment regimen did not increase the postural fall significantly except in the patients receiving a β-adrenoceptor blocking drug as the major part of the regimen. When the established dose of prazosin was reduced by one-third for a week, blood pressure rose by $15/8 \pm 12/9$mm Hg in the supine position, whilst erect pressure rose by $17/11 \pm 9/11$mm Hg. In a subsequent report by Simpson (1977b) involving 48 patients treated for an average period of 3 months, most of whom had prazosin added because of inadequate response to other drugs, it was noted that blood pressure was reduced by 20/15 and 25/17mm Hg in the supine and erect positions respectively.

A reduction in diastolic blood pressure (in any position) to 100mm Hg or less was achieved by Hayes et al. (1976a, 1977) in 38 of 50 patients, most of whom (45) were also receiving combined therapy with other antihypertensive drugs. The most common combination was prazosin, a β-adrenoceptor blocking drug and a diuretic. In 44 patients prazosin was introduced because of an inadequate response to, or side effects from, other drugs. The blood pressure of the whole group of 50 patients was reduced by an average of 31/20mm Hg (from 184/120 to 153/100mm Hg) during an average duration of therapy of 6.6 months. Hypertensive cardiac disease and renal impairment did not influence response to prazosin and the need for maintenance haemodialysis therapy and renal transplantation did not preclude its administration, negate an adequate response or produce an increased incidence of side effects.

A combination of prazosin, propranolol and a diuretic was effective in reducing blood pressure to normotensive levels in 22 of 25 patients, treated by Martinez et al. (1978), whose blood pressure had failed to respond to other combinations of drugs.

A satisfactory response (not defined) was reported in 47 (67%) of 70 patients who were treated with prazosin in doses of up to 30mg daily in addition to existing therapy in an attempt to improve control of blood pressure (Hua et al., 1976). The mean falls in blood pressure in these patients, whose serum creatinine was lower than 0.2mmol/L (approx. 2.27mg/100ml) was 36/24mm Hg supine and 32/22mm Hg erect. There was no significant alteration in doses of other antihypertensive agents before and after the use of prazosin. Another 10 patients initially had a satisfactory response to the addition of prazosin but blood pressure control later became unsatisfactory and an increased dose of prazosin or the addition of other agents was necessary. 3 patients admitted to not taking their drugs regularly. Three responded to an increased dose of propranolol and others to the addition of hydrallazine 75mg daily. 10 patients were given prazosin because of side effects from other antihypertensive drugs. Side effects complained of previously disappeared in 8 of these patients. Adequate control of blood pressure was also achieved and maintained in 10 of 24 patients with serum creatinine levels above 0.2mmol/L; mean falls in blood pressure in these 10 patients were 50.9/34.7mm Hg supine and 60.3/36mm Hg erect. There were no simultaneous changes in other antihypertensive treatment.

Turner et al. (1975) reported that the addition of prazosin to other antihypertensive therapy, which included debrisoquine, thiazide, clonidine or a β-adrenoceptor blocking drug alone or in various combinations, reduced the average supine blood pressure from 186/115mm Hg to 150/90 in 13 patients. Erect blood pressure was reduced from 205/110mm Hg to 133/85mm Hg. Turner et al. (1977) further reported that the addition of prazosin (mean dose 7mg daily) to existing antihypertensive therapy in 50 patients (35 WHO stage II or III) resulted in a reduction of erect diastolic blood pressure to below 90mm Hg in 36 patients (72%). In another 26 patients (16 stage II or III) in whom a mean reduction of 17/14mm Hg was achieved with prazosin alone, the addition of other drugs (β-blocker in 12; β-blocker plus thiazide in 14) resulted in a further mean reduction of 25/14mm Hg and normalisation of blood pressure in 19 patients (73%). 20 of 24 patients (15 stage I) became normotensive with prazosin alone (mean 6.5mg daily).

In a report on 100 patients (mostly with severe hypertension) in whom blood pressure had not responded adequately to previous therapy (Stokes et al., 1977a), the addition of prazosin resulted in a satisfactory response in 63% of patients. The response rate in the 78 followed for longer than 6 months was 73%. The average fall in blood pressure in these patients was 30/22mm Hg. A fall in blood pressure of at least 30/10mm Hg was achieved in 15 of 24 patients when prazosin (up to 30mg daily) was added to other drugs (diuretic, propranolol, clonidine in most) which had failed to control blood pressure. Those who failed to respond had more severe target organ damage than those who responded (Lubbe, 1977).

A 20% average reduction in blood pressure in 10 patients with hypertension refractory to previous therapy was obtained when hydrallazine 150 to 200mg daily in the previous regimen was replaced by prazosin 4 to 15mg (Pape et al., 1977).

On the basis of present evidence it seems that prazosin is a useful addition to the treatment regimen of patients whose blood pressure is not satisfactorily controlled by combinations of other drugs with a different mode of action. In patients who fail to respond to such combinations within a few weeks of the inclusion of prazosin, the addition of hydrallazine or diazoxide, may be of benefit.

5.6 Prazosin in Patients with Renal Disease

In patients with impaired renal function elevated blood pressure is often difficult to treat and it is usually necessary to combine several antihypertensive agents to control the blood pressure (Kincaid-Smith and Hua, 1974). Prazosin has been added to the treatment regimen of several patients with impaired renal function with an improvement in blood pressure (Curtis and Bateman, 1975; Bailey et al., 1976; Bailey, 1977; Hayes et al., 1976; Hua et al., 1976); which may be the result of the additional administration of a drug with a different mechanism of action, rather than a unique effect of prazosin. At present, there is no evidence that the addition of prazosin to existing combined antihypertensive therapy resulted in further deterioration in residual renal function, a significant improvement being recorded by Hayes (1977) and by Bailey (1977) in some patients, particularly those in whom impairment was due to hypertension alone and the glomerular filtration only mildly to moderately reduced.

In the study of Hayes et al. (1976a), 28 of 50 patients had impaired renal function, some of whom required maintenance haemodialysis therapy and renal transplantation. Renal function impairment was not associated with a reduced response rate or an increased incidence of side effects.

Curtis and Bateman (1975) monitored renal function by means of ^{51}Cr-EDTA clearances, plasma creatinine and blood urea in 12 patients with chronic renal failure (7) or renal transplant (5) who were treated with prazosin (mean dose 3mg daily). Concomitant antihypertensive therapy was used in all patients; α-methyldopa, propranolol, clonidine and a diuretic were the other drugs most commonly used. More than one of these drugs was used along with prazosin in 9 patients. There was no significant difference in the blood urea concentration, plasma creatinine concentration or ^{51}Cr-EDTA clearances during the control and prazosin periods in the patients in whom these variables were measured. The average blood pressure for all patients before prazosin treatment was 194/120mm Hg supine and 187/119mm Hg erect. During prazosin treatment, the supine and erect pressures were 167/103 and

149/96mm Hg respectively. There was a significant fall in the erect systolic and diastolic pressures during prazosin but not during the control period, which suggested a greater postural effect when prazosin was added to the regimen.

A greater orthostatic component with prazosin as compared with α-methyldopa or propranolol was reported by Stokes and Weber (1974). An average dose of 7mg of prazosin produced satisfactory control of blood pressure in 29 of 35 patients with mild to moderate blood pressure and renal disease treated by Bailey (1977). Findings in 16 of these patients were reported by Bailey et al. (1976). As in the other studies in which renal function was evaluated during prazosin, there was no deterioration of renal function attributable to the drug.

Prazosin (mean dose 6.55mg daily) was given in conjunction with other antihypertensive therapy which had failed to adequately control blood pressure in 24 patients whose serum creatinine was above 0.2mmol/L (approx. 2.27mg/100ml). Blood pressure was controlled in 10 of the patients (Hua et al., 1976). There was no rise in serum creatinine levels above the values at the beginning of the study. A similar dosage of prazosin (mean 7mg) was associated with a mean fall in blood pressure of 28/22mm Hg in 29 patients treated by Bailey (1977).

Curtis (1974) noted that patients with chronic renal failure responded with a fall in blood pressure after low doses of prazosin, and recommended that small doses (i.e. < 2mg daily) be used initially in such patients. This observation is borne out in the study of Curtis and Bateman (1975) where the addition of a mean dose of 3mg/d prazosin to other antihypertensive therapy resulted in a significant fall in blood pressure in 12 patients with chronic renal failure (vide supra).

5.7 Rapid Lowering of Blood Pressure by Prazosin

Single large oral doses (mean 5.4mg)[3] have been used to lower blood pressure rapidly in small numbers of patients with hypertension following renal biopsy, renovascular surgery and renal transplantation, during peritoneal dialysis and in patients with severe hypertension (Hayes, 1977). A reduction of diastolic blood pressure by 20mm Hg or to 100mm Hg was achieved on 7 of 11 occasions when the response was measured at 60 to 120 minutes and on 11 of 12 occasions when the response was determined at 180 to 240 minutes. Patients who failed to respond to single large oral doses of prazosin were those receiving the drug as maintenance antihypertensive therapy.

3   In the USA, single initial doses exceeding 1mg (capsules) are not recommended.

6. Factors Influencing Response to Prazosin

6.1 Dosage

There is a clearly increased antihypertensive effect in most patients when a thiazide diuretic is added to prazosin (section 5.3) and when prazosin is added to existing antihypertensive therapy (section 5.5), although an increase in antihypertensive effect resulting from an increase in the dosage of prazosin when used as the sole antihypertensive agent has been less clearly demonstrated, probably because dosage has not been increased beyond an arbitrary chosen maximum. In terms of response rate, there is an increased percentage response with an increase in dosage (Pitts, 1975).

Amery et al. (1974) found that prazosin 3mg daily produced only an insignificant reduction in blood pressure measured in the clinic in 23 patients with mild to moderate essential hypertension. An increase in the dose of prazosin to 7.5mg daily in 15 of these patients resulted in a significant fall in supine and diastolic blood pressure recorded at home. Only diastolic home blood pressure was significantly reduced by 3mg daily and then to a somewhat lesser extent.

An improvement in blood pressure upon increasing the dose of prazosin from 3 to 7.5mg daily was noted by Stokes and Weber (1974) in 4 of 9 patients so treated but it was not possible to dissociate improvement due to increased dosage from that possibly due to a delayed maximum effect or to the introduction of diuretic treatment.

A combination of prazosin and polythiazide was used in all 20 patients treated by Oh et al. (1975), the dosage of prazosin being increased at 4-week intervals. No further reduction in blood pressure was achieved by increasing the dosage of prazosin above 15mg daily despite the fact that diastolic blood pressure was still above 90mm Hg in half of the patients.

In a multicentre study, Thulin et al. (1974) reported a significant reduction in diastolic blood pressure in 30 patients treated with 6mg daily of prazosin, an effect which was maintained during a further observation period (mean 20 weeks) in 16 of these patients. Increasing the dosage to 15mg daily did not further reduce the blood pressure in the 12 patients followed up for 25 weeks. Venables and Duff (1974) increased the dosage from 3mg to 6mg daily in 7 patients who responded poorly to the lower dose. A more marked fall was recorded in 2 patients, the fall continued along the same gradient as initially in 1 and decreased in 4.

Results of 2 studies (Okun, 1974) which compared the same total daily dosage of prazosin given in divided doses twice, three or four times daily, suggest that frequency of administration is not critical. A similar degree of blood pressure control might be expected, once the optimum dosage has been reached, whether prazosin is given twice, three, or four times daily.

In most of these studies, results for individual patients have not been given and it is certain that some patients would have benefited from an increase in the dosage of prazosin. However, a moderate reduction in the blood pressure of a few patients may

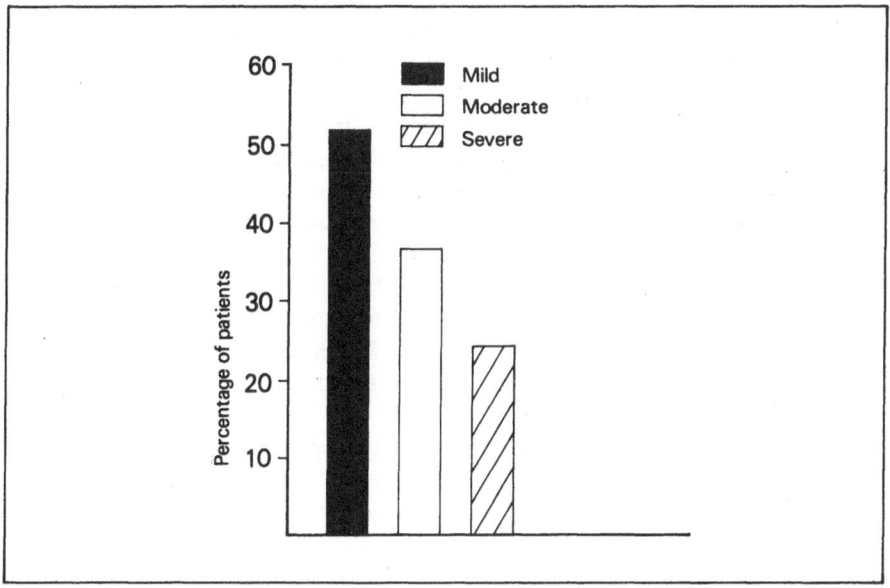

Fig. 3. Percentage of patients with mild, moderate or severe hypertension whose supine diastolic blood pressure was reduced to 90mm Hg or below during treatment with prazosin.

not influence the average blood pressure for a study group as a whole and thus the lack of change recorded in some studies may mask the response in individual patients. However, the benefit of adding a thiazide to prazosin in those who fail to respond to moderate doses of the drug is clearly evident in several studies and it would appear wise to use a prazosin-thiazide regimen in preference to increasing the dose of prazosin alone in initial non-responders in an attempt to control their blood pressure.

6.2 Baseline Severity of Blood Pressure, and Impaired Renal Function

As might be expected, there has been a tendency for prazosin used as the sole antihypertensive agent to lower diastolic blood pressure to 'normal' (< 90mm Hg) more frequently in patients with mild or moderate hypertension than in those with severe hypertension (fig. 3). In most studies which have used 15mg or more daily of prazosin (e.g. Bradley, 1975; Cohen, 1970; Feng et al., 1976; Kim, 1976; de la Pas et al., 1975; Pitkajarvi et al., 1977; Rab and Farooqui, 1975) the trend towards a better response in mild to moderate disease has been evident. Bradley (1974) reported that supine diastolic blood pressure was reduced to 90mm Hg or less in 16 of 24 patients with mild hypertension, in 8 of 19 with moderate disease and in none of 3 with severe disease. Similarly, normalisation of blood pressure in patients with mild,

moderate or severe to gross hypertension[4] was achieved by Cohen (1970) in 4 of 12,
5 of 14 and none of 12 respectively. De la Pas added polythiazide to prazosin therapy
in patients whose blood pressure was not adequately controlled by 20mg daily of
prazosin alone. Polythiazide was added to the treatment regimen in 5 of 6, 4 of 16
and none of 7, with severe, moderate and mild disease respectively.

However, such a clear trend has not been present in all studies. In the study of
Hayes et al. (1976a) the mean baseline diastolic pressure (117mm Hg) of patients who
responded to prazosin therapy was only slightly lower than that (125mm Hg) of those
who failed to respond. Stokes and Weber (1974) reported a satisfactory response in 3
of 6 patients with moderate hypertension and in 6 of 8 with severe disease. In an open
study in Argentina by Zapala and Bengolea (1973), the diastolic blood pressure was
reduced to 90mm Hg or below in all 11 patients with severe or gross hypertension
and in 2 of 3 with moderate hypertension.

Patients with chronic renal failure appear to respond with a significant fall in
blood pressure to a relatively low dose of prazosin (Curtis and Bateman, 1975) and
small doses should be used initially in such patients (see also section 4).

6.3 Duration of Therapy

The apparent lack of response to given doses of prazosin in some studies (e.g.
Amery et al., 1974; Cohen, 1970; Schirger and Sheps, 1977) may have been due in
part to the short duration on any particular treatment regimen. A delay of about 6
weeks before the full effects of a given dosage of prazosin become evident has been
reported by some investigators (Kuokkanen and Mattila, 1975; Lee and Seo, 1975;
Mroczek and Finnerty, 1974; Stokes and Weber, 1974).

Just as the full effect of prazosin may not be apparent for several weeks, the hypotensive effect of the drug may continue for a few weeks after it has been withdrawn. This carry-over effect is demonstrated in the study of Kuokkanen and Mattila
(1975) in which polythiazide was given in place of prazosin to 10 outpatients who
had received prazosin alone for the previous 6 weeks. A statistically significant
further fall in standing blood pressure occurred for the first 2 weeks after polythiazide
was substituted for prazosin. Blood pressure rose again during the fifth and sixth
weeks on polythiazide alone. However, Bolli and Simpson (1975) found a considerable rise in blood pressure one week after reduction of the dose of prazosin by
one-third.

---

4   'Gross' hypertension defined as 130mm Hg and above, diastolic; 'severe' hypertension as 115 to
129mm Hg diastolic.

7. What is the Role of Prazosin in the Treatment of Hypertension?

Prazosin has been shown in adequately designed studies to be an effective antihypertensive drug when used alone (section 5.1) and in combination with a thiazide diuretic (section 5.3) or other antihypertensive drugs (section 5.4).

It is effective in lowering blood pressure in all grades of hypertension: when used alone in mild and some cases of moderate severity, or in combination with other agents in moderate to severe cases. When given in combination with a thiazide diuretic it is generally effective in controlling blood pressure in a high proportion of patients with severe as well as moderate hypertension. It may be particularly useful as an adjunct to existing antihypertensive therapy in patients who are unable to tolerate further dose increments of these drugs or in whom blood pressure is not adequately controlled by them (e.g. Hua et al., 1976).

As prazosin and β-adrenoceptor blocking drugs have a different mode of action and augment each others antihypertensive effect (Marshall et al., 1977) their combined use, perhaps also with a thiazide diuretic, is a logical and an effective regimen in the treatment of severe hypertension. Prazosin may also be used as a substitute for hydrallazine as it appears to cause fewer troublesome side effects and to be equipotent with hydrallazine in a ratio of 1 to 20 or 30mg (Kincaid-Smith, 1975, Kincaid-Smith et al., 1977; Rassmussen and Jensen, 1975, 1976, 1977; section 5.4). In occasional cases prazosin (because of its different mode of action) in addition to low doses of hydrallazine may be useful when used with other drugs in the treatment of resistant hypertension (Hua et al., 1976).

Prazosin is effective in newly diagnosed hypertensive patients, particularly when used in combination with a thiazide diuretic. Polythiazide 2 to 4mg daily has been used in most studies so far. Although in many studies a thiazide has not been added until the maximum dosage (usually 20mg/day) of prazosin has been reached, there is some evidence (Cohen, 1970; Maher, 1975; Oh et al., 1974; Oviasu and Idahosa, 1976; Paul et al., 1976; Rougier et al., 1974) that earlier introduction of the thiazide may produce equally satisfactory blood pressure control with a lower dosage or prazosin in some patients. Thus, on the basis of present data it seems that the thiazide diuretic of the physician's choice can be used initially, or alternatively should be introduced once some response to moderate doses of prazosin is apparent and then the dosage of prazosin gradually increased if necessary. In clinical practice, many patients would already be receiving treatment with a diuretic before being given prazosin.

Studies in patients with renal disease and impairment (section 5.5) indicate that the addition of prazosin to existing antihypertensive therapy does not result in deterioration of remaining renal function. Although long term studies in large numbers of patients with renal impairment are needed to determine the effects, if any, of prazosin in such patients, present evidence suggests that prazosin can be successfully used in low doses in patients with chronic renal failure. It should be borne in mind that Curtis (1974) and Curtis and Bateman (1975) found patients with chronic renal failure to be particularly responsive to low dosages of prazosin; the drug should therefore be introduced cautiously in low dosages (1 to 2mg daily).

As prazosin does not increase serum uric acid or blood sugar levels and is effective in many patients without added thiazide therapy, it is suitable for use in patients with gout or diabetes mellitus (Kincaid-Smith et al., 1973).

The development of tolerance has not been clearly documented and in most long term studies has not been evident (Melkild, 1977; Moyer, 1975; Okun, 1975; Stokes et al., 1977; Zapala and Bengolea, 1973). The need to increase the dosage of prazosin or to add other therapy to maintain satisfactory control was reported by Hua et al. (1976) and Seedat et al. (1975a). The reason for the loss of blood pressure control after an initially satisfactory response was not clear in most of the patients. Mabadeje (1978) reported that 16 of 40 patients developed tolerance to the antihypertensive effect of prazosin, but its development was not defined.

As prazosin does not decrease cardiac output, it could be expected to be useful in patients with hypertension and Raynauds phenomenon (Lund-Johansen, personal communication). On the other hand, as prazosin has no significant effect on the heart rate, and thus relatively less effect on the systolic pressure-heart rate product, the drug is less suitable for patients with hypertension and angina pectoris (see also section 8.4). In such patients β-adrenoceptor blocking drugs which markedly reduce both heart rate and pressure may have advantages.

8. Side Effects

At dosages usually given for the control of hypertension, prazosin has been relatively well tolerated by most patients and only occasionally has it been necessary to discontinue the drug because of adverse effects. Dizziness and faintness, usually associated with postural hypotension, have been the most commonly reported effects. There has been a tendency for adverse effects to be more frequent during the initial treatment period and to decrease as treatment continued, irrespective of the daily dose required to control blood pressure. However, the incidence of postural effects appears to be related to the dose given initially (or to an excessively rapid dose increment), although these effects usually disappear as treatment continues.

8.1 Postural Effects

Adverse effects described as dizziness and faintness have been reported by many investigators. In the studies reporting such effects their incidence during the initial stages of treatment has ranged from about 7% (Research Group, Japan, 1977) to

58 % (Stokes and Weber, 1974; Turner, 1976a,b). It is not certain whether or not the dizziness and allied effects reported in all studies are associated with a fall in standing blood pressure as in only some studies have blood pressure measurements been reported during the time that these effects have been present. Dizziness does not appear to be related to abnormally high plasma levels of prazosin (Graham et al., 1976b; Simpson et al., 1977; Verbesselt et al., 1976).

In several studies the postural effects have been associated with syncope and appear to be related to the initial dosage (Gabriel et al., 1975a,b; Seedat et al., 1975b; Rees and Williams, 1975; Rosendorff, 1976; Turner, 1976a,b) and to occur most often with the first dose (Verbesselt et al., 1976; Graham et al., 1976b). Intensive monitoring and follow-up of the first 23,000 patients in the United States of America receiving prazosin 1 mg (as capsules) 3 times daily as a starting dose indicated an incidence of 0.15 % (34 confirmed cases) of syncope (Norris, 1977, personal communication).

In two studies in which prazosin tablets were used (Rosendorff 1976; Turner, 1976a,b), patients who reacted with postural symptoms to the first dose of 1 or 2mg prazosin were rechallenged at a later date with a single 0.5mg dose. None of the 14 patients who experienced significant postural hypotension when given 1mg prazosin as the first dose, experienced adverse symptoms when given a dose of 0.5mg (Turner, 1976a). Similarly, in the study of Rosendorff (1976), only 2 of 7 who entered the rechallenge study after having experienced postural symptoms at a first dose of 2mg, reported symptoms after a 0.5mg dose. Graham et al. (1976b) reported postural hypotension after an initial 2mg dose (tablets) of prazosin in 6 patients, but that these effects dissipated during 2 days of continuous treatment, despite higher plasma levels, and were barely significant on subsequent challenge with a 2mg dose. Appreciable, though less severe 'first dose' effects occurred after a dose of 0.5mg (tablets) in another group of 3 patients.

In the studies which have specifically studied the 'first dose' effect, the symptoms of postural hypotension occurred within 3 hours of the first dose and in the studies of Graham et al. (1976b), Simpson (1977b) and Turner (1976a) were accompanied by documented pronounced falls in standing blood pressure. The mean fall in standing blood pressure was 63/48mm Hg in those with symptoms, compared with 22/14mm Hg in those who did not experience symptoms of postural hypotension. Verbesselt et al. (1976) found that 2 fasted normal subjects who experienced marked postural hypotension after a single 2mg dose (tablets) of prazosin did not experience this effect when given the same dose 2 and 4 days later with food, or when given 0.5, 1 and 2mg (tablets) doses in the fasted state two weeks later. An interval of 1 week was allowed between each rechallenge dose. The presence of food did not reduce the prazosin serum levels in these subjects.

The postural hypotensive reaction may be peculiar only to the first dose of the drug in some patients and rechallenge, even with the same dose, may not result in a recurrence of the reaction. However, postural effects may also occur following rapid increases in dosage (Bailey et al., 1976; Simpson 1977b; Stokes et al., 1977; Turner et al., 1977) and in some patients may persist beyond the first few doses (Marshall et al., 1977; Simpson, 1977b; Stokes et al., 1977).

Results of a recent study of 'first dose' effects of prazosin by Graham et al. (1976b) suggests that postural effects may be more severe in patients on a low sodium diet and concomitant therapy with β-adrenoceptor blocking drugs and might be expected in patients who may be relatively sodium depleted as a result of previous diuretic treatment. In such patients marked falls in blood pressure may accompany initial doses as low as 0.25mg (tablets) [Simpson et al., 1977]. A further study (Stokes, et al., 1977) of the influence of dietary sodium on the 'first dose' effects of prazosin suggests that orthostatic symptoms are less likely during a sodium intake of 250mEq daily, and that increased dietary sodium may be as effective as dosage reduction in preventing 'first dose' hypotensive responses.

Thus it seems from the limited rechallenge studies that have been conducted that 'first dose' postural hypotension may be largely avoided by beginning treatment with a low dose in the region of 0.5mg twice daily (tablets) or 1mg 3 times daily (capsules) with the first dose given at bedtime. It is also possible that this effect may be confined to the first dose of the drug in many patients. However, it seems advisable to start the first few days of treatment with low doses, particularly in patients who are already receiving a diuretic and/or β-adrenoceptor blocking drugs or who may be relatively sodium depleted as a result of previous diuretic therapy.

8.2 Changes in Heart Rate

Prazosin, unlike hydrallazine, usually does not cause a rise in heart rate. Any increase in heart rate caused by prazosin is generally mild to moderate and more apparent in the erect position (e.g. Fernandes et al., 1975; Falase et al., 1976). It is possible that the lack of effect on heart rate in some studies may be due to the failure to monitor the heart rate in the standing as well as in the supine position, although few studies have reported significant changes in heart rate. In a study in which heart rate was monitored by ECG at rest and sitting, long term therapy with prazosin did not induce any significant changes in heart rate in either position (Lund-Johansen, 1974).

Palpitations have been reported occasionally (Bailey, 1977; Bendall et al., 1975; Bloom et al., 1975; Koukkanen and Mattilda, 1975; Oviasu and Idahosa, 1976; Paul et al., 1976; Seedat et al., 1975a; Simpson, 1977b; Thulin et al., 1974; Verhiest et al., 1974), but have not always been associated with a clear rise in heart rate (e.g. Kuokkanen and Mattila, 1975). In some instances palpitations have been associated with postural effects (Bendall et al., 1975; Seedat et al., 1975a) and syncope (Seedat et al., 1975b).

Tachycardia has occurred infrequently, although in two studies (Bendall et al., 1975; Bolli and Simpson, 1975) prazosin was given with other drugs and in some instances (Bailey, 1976; Bendall et al., 1975) tachycardia was associated with symptoms of postural hypotension. The heart rate response to exercise has been reported to be normal during exercise levels at 50, 100 and 150 watt (Lund-Johansen, 1974).

8.3 Skin Reactions

Skin eruptions or lesions have been reported on rare occasions and have not been clearly associated with the use of prazosin (Curtis and Bateman, 1975; Lund-Johansen, 1974).

An erythema nodosum-like eruption after 5 weeks' prazosin was reported by Curtis and Bateman (1975) in a patient also receiving clonidine, chlorothiazide and propranolol. The skin reaction failed to improve after withdrawal of the thiazide, then prazosin, but slow improvement occurred after cessation of propranolol.

A skin rash resembling lupus erythematosus occurred after 18 months on prazosin in a patient treated by Lund-Johansen (1974). Biopsy indicated that lupus erythematosus was likely. A generalised outbreak 6 weeks after prazosin was replaced by a β-adrenoceptor blocking drug (atenolol), responded to hydroxychloroquine without withdrawal of the β-adrenoceptor blocking drug. Antinuclear factor was negative and it was thought unlikely that the reaction was related to the drugs. The patient has continued on the same β-blocking drug for 3 years. He has had no more generalised outbreaks, but two exacerbations of his skin eruption following exposure to sunlight (Lund-Johansen 1977, personal communication).

8.4 Other Effects

Other effects possibly associated with the use of prazosin include headache, lassitude, dry mouth, diarrhoea, weight gain (with peripheral oedema in one study; Falase et al., 1976), nausea, urinary frequency with urgency, dry mouth, irritability, mental depression, ankle swelling, nasal stuffiness, constipation, acute febrile polyarthritis (Cairns and Jordan, 1976) and eosinophilia (Verhiest et al., 1974). As a side effect check list was used in some studies it is difficult to determine whether or not the reported effects are really associated with the use of prazosin. Transient deterioration of renal function during combined prazosin and propranolol therapy was reported by Curtis and Bateman (1975), but was considered to be associated with severe postural hypotension.

Angina pectoris has been reported to be aggravated by the use of prazosin in Australasia (Kellaway, 1976; Raftos, 1976; Simpson, 1977b; Stokes et al., 1977) but in the experience of Turner (personal communication, 1977) angina has not been aggravated or produced as a new symptom since low doses of prazosin have been used

Table VI. Incidence of side effects in double-blind studies in hypertensive patients treated with prazosin or α-methyldopa

Authors	No. of pats.	No. of side effects							
		Prazosin[1]				α-Methyldopa			
		PD	H	Other	Dis	PD	H	Other	Dis
Bloom et al. (1975)	30	2	4	13	4	1	4	13	0
Bradley et al. (1977)	45	1	0	14	0	2	3	14	1
Mroczek and Finnerty (1974)	42	4	3	6	0	3	5	5	0
Schnaper and Oberman (1975)	39	,12	14	57	0	5	10	49	2

1 Abbreviations: PD = postural dizziness; H = headache; Dis = therapy discontinued due to side effects.

to initiate therapy. In one of these patients the symptoms were probably a reflection of the lack of response of blood pressure to therapy (Bolli and Simpson, 1974).

Other factors could also have contributed to the angina, such as a reduction in the dosage of concomitant β-adrenoceptor blocking therapy (Simpson, 1977b). Angina pectoris was associated with faintness after taking glyceryl trinitrate in one patient treated by Stokes et al. (1977), whilst in 2 further patients the symptoms were controlled by verapamil and prazosin therapy was continued (Stokes et al., 1977). A myocardial infarction rate of 1 episode per 185 patient months was noted by Simpson et al. (1977) during prazosin therapy but this may be a reasonable rate in a group of patients in the age range of 55 to 73 years. However, it is considered that prazosin may produce angina pectoris as a new symptom (Kellaway, 1976) and its use may be associated with myocardial infarction (Simpson et al., 1977), but it is not clear whether or not these symptoms are definitely related to the use of prazosin. It must also be remembered that excessive reduction of blood pressure with any antihypertensive drug can result in symptoms of cerebrovascular insufficiency or angina and may even precipitate cerebrovascular accidents or myocardial infarction.

8.5 Incidence of Side Effects Compared with α-Methyldopa

In studies which have compared the incidence of side effects in the same or parallel groups of patients under the controlled conditions of therapeutic trials (table VI; fig. 4), the total number of side effects have been very similar. Whilst it appears that prazosin may not cause some of the effects (e.g. positive Coombs' test; impotence) associated with the long term use of α-methyldopa, the pattern of side effects in trials comparing prazosin and α-methyldopa has not indicated that overall they are more of a problem with α-methyldopa over periods of 12 weeks to 8 months.

In many anecdotal reports which suggest that side effects are less of a problem with prazosin than with α-methyldopa, there has probably been a tendency for investigators to compare the effects noted over the few weeks of the trial of prazosin with those known to occur with α-methyldopa when given over a more prolonged period. Schnaper and Oberman (1974) reported a total of 83 side effects in 20 patients treated for 6 weeks with prazosin, and 64 side effects over the same period in 19 patients treated with α-methyldopa. Mroczek and Finnerty (1974) reported a total of 13 side effects with both prazosin and α-methyldopa at dosages required to control blood pressure. Similarly, Bloom et al. (1975) reported 19 side effects in 25 patients receiving prazosin and 18 of 27 patients given α-methyldopa. A somewhat lower overall incidence of side effects was reported by Venables and Duff (1974) who recorded 4 side effects with prazosin and 6 with α-methyldopa.

Thus, on the basis of results of controlled comparative trials there is no difference in the overall incidence of side effects with therapeutically equivalent doses of prazosin and α-methyldopa. Drowsiness or tiredness has tended to be more frequent with α-methyldopa, and postural dizziness more common with prazosin. However, the dizziness associated with prazosin is usually only temporary whilst that with α-methyldopa tends to persist. It has not been indicated if the headaches seen with

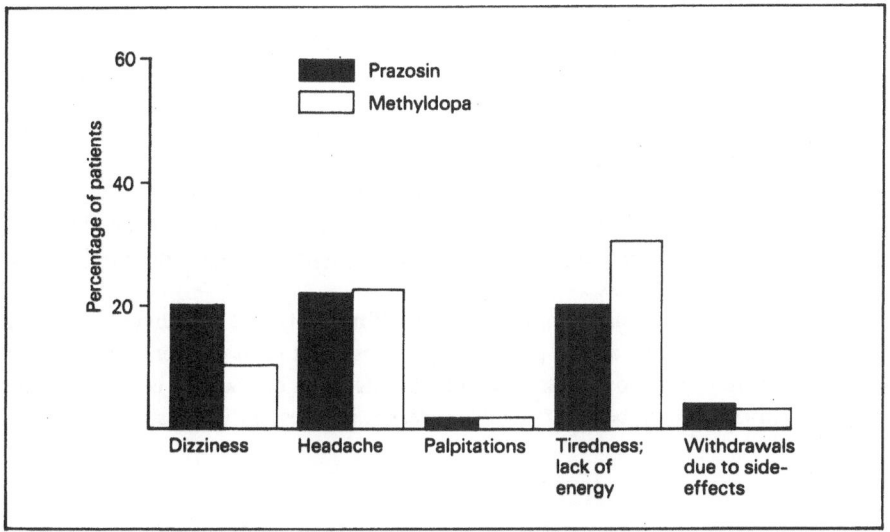

Fig. 4. Percentage of hypertensive patients who experienced certain side effects in controlled comparisons of prazosin and α-methyldopa (data from studies of Bloom et al., 1975; Bradley et al., 1977; Mroczek and Finnerty, 1974; Schnaper and Oberman 1975).

prazosin are of the vascular type often seen with higher doses of hydrallazine. A major advantage of prazosin is its freedom from effects on sexual function.

8.6 Incidence of Side effects Compared with Hydrallazine

Results of double-blind trials comparing equiactive antihypertensive doses of prazosin and hydrallazine in combination with a thiazide and β-adrenoceptor blocking drug, indicate that side effects are more of a problem with hydrallazine than with prazosin (Kincaid-Smith, 1975; 1977). Whereas side effects necessitated the withdrawal of hydrallazine in 7 patients, only 1 patient discontinued prazosin because of adverse effects.

9. Precautions

Syncope with sudden loss of consciousness may occur, usually within 30 to 90 minutes of an excessive initial dose of prazosin (sections 8.1; 10). More common than loss of consciousness are the symptoms of dizziness and lightheadedness associated with the initial lowering of blood pressure. Patients should be warned to avoid situations where injury could result should syncope occur during the initiation of prazosin therapy.

10. Dosage

As some patients experience severe postural hypotensive symptoms with the initial or first few doses of prazosin it is essential to begin treatment with a low dose; e.g. 0.5mg as tablets 2 or 3 times daily or 1mg 3 times daily as capsules.* As this dose is intended primarily to minimise 'first dose' reactions, the dosage should be increased gradually from the first return visit. Some suggest a minimum of 3 days between each dosage increase.

The usual dosage range of prazosin is 3 to 20mg daily in 2 or 3 divided doses. A few patients may require and respond to higher doses but most workers prefer to add a thiazide diuretic once some response to moderate doses of prazosin is apparent, the dosage of prazosin then being gradually increased if necessary (see also sections 6.1;

---

* In the USA, prazosin is available as capsules. The initial dosage recommendation with this dose form is different from the tablets because the capsule formulation results in lower peak plasma levels of prazosin.

7). Following initial dose titration of prazosin some patients can be maintained adequately on a twice daily dosage regimen.

When a thiazide diuretic or other antihypertensive agent is added the dosage of prazosin should be reduced (e.g. halved) and subsequently adjusted as required to obtain an adequate response (see also section 5.5).

A period of 4 to 6 weeks may be required for the full antihypertensive effect to become apparent, thus an adequate time should be allowed for the response to become optimum before increasing the dose. Response is usually seen within 1 to 14 days if it is to occur at any particular dose. When a response is seen treatment should be continued at that dose until the degree of response has reached the optimum before the next dose increment.

Acknowledgements

Various sections of the manuscript reviewed by: *A. Amery*, Department of Medicine, Academisch Ziekenhuis Sint-Rafael, Belgium; *J.R. Curtis*, Charing Cross Hospital, London, England; *R.W. Gifford*, The Cleveland Clinic Foundation, Cleveland, Ohio, USA; *F. Gross*, Department of Pharmacology, University of Heidelberg, Federal Republic of Germany; *L.I. Goldberg*, Department of Pharmacological and Physiological Sciences, The University of Chicago, Illinois, USA; *Priscilla Kincaid-Smith*, Department of Medicine, Royal Melbourne Hospital, Victoria, Australia; *P. Lund-Johansen*, Department of Medicine, University of Bergen School of Medicine, Norway; *M. Moser*, Davis Avenue Medical Centre, White Plains, New York, U.S.A.; *G. Onesti*, Division of Nephrology and Hypertension, Hahnemann, Medical College, Philadelphia, USA; *J.S. Peel*, Hawke's Bay Medical Research Foundation, Napier, New Zealand; *J.I.S. Robertson*, Medical Research Council Blood Pressure Unit, Western Infirmary, Glasgow, Scotland; *F.O. Simpson*, Department of Medicine, University of Otago, Dunedin, New Zealand; *P. Sleight*, Department of Cardiovascular Medicine, Radcliffe Infirmary, Oxford, England. *G.S. Stokes*, Medical Research Department, Sydney Hospital, Australia; *A.S. Turner*, Cardiology Department, Napier Hospital, New Zealand.

References

Amery, A.; Verhiest, W.; Crooneberghs, J. and Fagard, R.: Double-blind crossover study with a new vasodilator — prazosin — in the treatment of mild hypertension. Hypovase Symposium, Geneva (March 1974).

Bailey, R.R.: The kidney and antihypertensive therapy. Drugs 11 (Suppl. 1): 70 (1976).

Bailey, R.R.: Prazosin in the treatment of patients with hypertension and renal function impairment. Special Supplement to the Medical Journal of Australia 2: 42 (1977).

Bailey, R.R.; Lynn, K.L.; Neale, T.L. and Little, P.J.: Prazosin in the treatment of patients with hypertension and renal function impairment. New Zealand Medical Journal 84: 467 (1967).

Bendall, M.J.; Baloch, K.H.; Wilson, P.R.: Side-effects due to treatment of hypertension with prazosin. British Medical Journal 2: 727 (1975).

Bianchetti, G.; Graziani, G.; Brancaccio, D.; Morganti, A.; Leonetti, G.; Manfrin, M.; Sega, R.; Gomeni, R.; Ponticelli, G. and Morselli, P.L.: Pharmacokinetics and effects of propranolol in terminal uraemic patients and in patients undergoing regular dialysis treatment. Clinical Pharmacokinetics 1: 373 (1976).

Bloom, D.S.; Rosendorff, C. and Kramer, R.: Clinical evaluation of prazosin as the sole agent for the treatment of hypertension: A double-blind crossover study with methyldopa. Current Therapeutic Research 18 (1): 144 (1975).

Bolli, P. and Simpson, F.O.: A preliminary clinical trial of prazosin: a new oral antihypertensive agent. New Zealand Medical Journal 79: 969 (1974).

Bolli, P. and Simpson, F.O.: Experience with prazosin in the treatment of hypertension. Postgraduate Medicine (Suppl. Nov): 69 (1975).

Bolli, P.; Wood, A.J.; Phelan, E.L.; Lee, D.R. and Simpson, F.O.: Prazosin: preliminary clinical and pharmacological observations. Clinical Science and Molecular Medicine 48: 177S (1975).

Bolli, P.; Wood, A.J. and Simpson, F.O.: Effects of prazosin in patients with hypertension. Clinical Pharmacology and Therapeutics 20: 138 (1976).

Bolzano, K.: Prazosin, a new quinazoline derivative in the treatment of essential hypertension. In Cotton (Ed) Prazosin — Evolution of a new antihypertensive agent (Excerpta Medica, Amsterdam 1974).

Bradley, W.F.: A long-term clinical trial of prazosin. Postgraduate Medicine (Suppl. Nov): 95 (1975).

Bradley, W.F.: Hoffman, F.G.; Hutchison, J.C.; Kalams, Z. and Waldron, S.L.: Comparison of prazosin and methyldopa in mild to moderate hypertension, a multicenter cooperative study. Current Therapeutic Research 21: 28 (1977).

Cairns, S.A. and Jordan, S.C.: Prazosin treatment complicated by acute febrile polyarthritis. British Medical Journal 2: 1424 (1976).

Cambridge, D.; Davey, M.J. and Massingham, R.: Prazosin, a selective antagonist of post-synaptic α-adrenoceptors. British Journal of Pharmacology 59: 514P (1977a).

Cambridge, D.; Davey, M.J. and Massingham, R.: The pharmacology of antihypertensive drugs with special reference to vasodilators, α-adrenergic blocking agents and prazosin. Medical Journal of Australia 2 (Suppl.): 2 (1977b).

Cambridge, D.; Davey, M.J. and Massingham, R.: Further evidence for a selective postsynaptic α-adrenoceptor blockade with prazosin in vascular smooth muscle. Nauyn-Schmeideberg's Archives of Pharmacology 302 (Suppl.) Abstract 206 (1978).

Cavero, I.: Cardiovascular effects of prazosin in dogs. Clinical Science and Molecular Medicine 57: 609S (1976).

Cavero, I.; Fenard, S.; Gomeni, R.; Lefevre, F. and Roach, A.G.: Studies on the mechanism of the vasodilator effects of prazosin in dogs and rabbits. European Journal of pharmacology 49: 259 (1978).

Cavero, I. and Lefevre, F.: Cardiovascular effects of prazosin in spontaneously hypertensive rats (SHR). Clinical and Experimental Pharmacology and Physiology 4 (Suppl. 3): 61 (1977).

Cavero, I.; Lefevre, F. and Roach, A.: Further studies on cardiovascular effects of prazosin. Federation Proceedings 36: 955 (1977a).

Cavero, I.; Lefevre, F. and Roach, A.G.: Differential effects of prazosin on the pre- and postsynaptic α-adrenoceptors in the rat and dog. British Journal of Pharmacology 61: 469p (1977b).

Cohen, B.M.: Prazosin hydrochloride (CP-12, 229-1), an oral antihypertensive agent: preliminary clinical observations in ambulatory patients. Journal of Clinical Pharmacology 10: 408 (1970).

Collier, J.G.; Lorge, R.E. and Robinson, B.F.: Comparison of effects tolmesoxide (RX 71107), diazoxide, hydrallazine, prazosin, glyceryl trinitrate and sodium nitroprusside on forearm arteries and dorsal hand veins of man. British Journal of Clinical Pharmacology 5: 35 (1978).

Collins, I.S. and Pek, P.: Pharmacokinetics of prazosin, a new antihypertensive compound. Clinical and Experimental Pharmacology and Physiology 2: 445 (1975).

Constantine, J.W.: Analysis of the hypertensive action of prazosin; in Cotton, (Ed) Prazosin — Evaluation of a new antihypertensive agent (Excerpta Medica, Amsterdam 1974).

Constantine, J.W.; McShane, W.K.; Scriabine, A. and Hess, H.J.: Analysis of the hypotensive action of prazosin. In Onesti, Kim and Moyer (Eds) Hypertension: Mechanisms and Management, p.449 (Grune and Stratton, New York 1973).

Curtis, J.R.: Prazosin in patients with chronic renal failure. British Medical Journal 3: 742 (1974).

Curtis, J.R. and Bateman, F.J.A.: Use of prazosin in management of hypertension in patients with chronic renal failure and renal transplant recipients. British Medical Journal 4: 432 (1975).

de la Paz, A.G.; Aquino, A. and Sawit, S.: Prazosin hydrochloride in the treatment of hypertension. Philippine Journal of Internal Medicine 3: 125 (1975).

de la Paz, A.G.; Reyes, A.L.; de Guia, R.; Saldivar, C.; Aquino, A.; Saniel, E.G.; Durante, M. and Unson, L.: A new quinazoline derivative in the treatment of hypertension. A co-operative study in four medical centres in the Philippines. Philippine Journal of Cardiology 4: 47 (1976).

England, J.D.; Trembath, P.W. and Shaw, J.: Plasma cyclic 3' 5' adenosine monophosphate (C'AMP) levels in hypertension: Effects of treatment. Abstract of paper presented at Annual Meeting of Australasian Society of Clinical and Experimental Pharmacologists, Adelaide, November 1976.

Falase, A.O.; Salako, L.A.; Aminu, J.M.: Lack of effect of low doses of prazosin in hypertensive Nigerians. Current Therapeutic Research 19: 603 (1976).

Feng, P.H.; Chan, H.C.; Tan, N.J. and Lee, Y.K.: Prazosin hydrochloride in the treatment of hypertension. Annals of the Academy of Medicine 5: 157 (1976).

Feng, P.H.; Ng, K.K.F.; Chan, H.C.; Tan, N.J. and Lee, Y.K.: Renin characterisation of hypertensive patients treated with vasodilation, beta-blockade and volume depletion. Annals of the Academy of Medicine, Singapore 4: 274 (1975).

Fernandes, M.; Smith, I.S.; Weder, A. et al.: Prazosin in the treatment of hypertension. Clinical Science and Molecular Medicine 48: 181S (1975).

Graham, R.M.; Muir, M.R. and Hayes, J.M.: Effects of prazosin on blood pressure and plasma renin activity in the anaesthetised dog. Australian and New Zealand Journal of Medicine 4: 424 (1974).

Graham, R.M.; Oates, H.F.; Stoker, I.M. and Stokes, G.S.: Mechanism of action of prazosin, an antihypertensive agent. Abstract of paper presented at Annual Meeting of Australasian Physiological and Pharmacological Society, Melbourne (August 1976a).

Graham, R.M.; Thornell, I.R.; Gain, J.M.; Bagnoli, C.; Oates, H.F. and Stokes, G.S.: Prazosin: the first-dose phenomenon. British Medical Journal 2: 1293 (1976b).

Graham, R.M.; Muir, M.R. and Hayes, J.M.: Differing effects of the vasodilator drugs, prazosin and diazoxide on plasma renin activity in the dog. Clinical and Experimental Pharmacology and Physiology 3: 193 (1976c).

Gabriel, R.; Meek, D. and Mamtora, H.: Adverse reactions to prazosin. Brit. med. J. 4: 41 (1975a).

Gabriel, R.; Meek, D. and Mamtora, H.: Adverse reactions to prazosin. Brit. med. J. 3: 41 (1975b).

Guevara-Viales, L.: Prazosin: New antihypertensive drug. Comparative study with α-methyldopa (translation). Revista Medica de Costa Rica 43: 11 (1976).

Hayes, J.M.: Prazosin in severe hypertension. Effect on blood pressure, plasma renin activity and in hypertensive emergencies. Medical Journal of Australia 2 (Suppl.): 30 (1977).

Hayes, J.M.; Graham, R.M.; O'Connell, B.P.; Speers, E. and Humphrey, T.J.: Effect of prazosin on plasma renin activity. Australian and New Zealand Journal of Medicine 6: 90 (1976b).

Hayes, J.M.; Graham, R.M.; O'Connell, B.P.; Speers, E. and Humphrey, T.J.: Experience with prazosin in the treatment of patients with severe hypertension. Medical Journal of Australia 1: 562 (1976a).

Hess, H.J.: Biochemistry and structure-activity studies with prazosin; in Cotton (Ed) Prazosin — Evaluation of a new antihypertensive agent. (Excerpta Medica, Amsterdam 1974).

Hobbs, D.C. and Twomey, T.M.: Pharmacokinetics of prazosin in man. Unpublished data (1977).

Hua, S.P.; MacDonald, Ileene M.; Myers, J.B. and Kincaid-Smith, P.: Studies with prazosin a new effective hypertensive agent. Medical Journal of Australia 1: 559 (1976).

Hua, A.S.P.; MacDonald, Ileene, M.: Myers, J.B.; Fang, P. and Kincaid-Smith, Priscilla: Studies with prazosin. A new effective hypotensive agent. II Two double-blind cross-over studies comparing the effects of prazosin and hydrallazine. Medical Journal of Australia 2: 5 (1977a)

Hua, A.S.P. and Moulds, R.F.W.: The effect of prazosin on pre- and post-synaptic α-adrenoceptors in the pithed rat. Australasian Society of Clinical and Experimental Pharmacologists Proceedings, Sydney (Nov. 1977b).

Hua, A.S.P.; Myers, J.B. and Kincaid-Smith, P.: Studies with prazosin — a new effective hypotensive agent. III An acute double-blind cross-over study comparing the effects of single doses of prazosin and hydrallazine in combination with propranolol and a diuretic. Medical Journal of Australia 1: 45 (1978).

Ibsen, H.; Rasmussen, K. and Herenlund, H.: Hendringer i plasma-volume, extracellulaervolumen og den glomerulaere filtrationshastighed under kombinationsbehandling med propranolol og prazosin has patienter med hypertension. Current Medical Research and Opinion 4 (Suppl. 2): 83 (1977).

Jauernig, R. and Moulds, R.F.W.: The use of isolated human arteries to study the action of prazosin and other hypotensive agents. Abstract of paper presented at Annual Meeting of Australasian Society of Clinical and Experimental Pharmacologists (November 1976).

Jauernig, R.A.; Moulds, R.F.W. and Shaw, J.: The action of prazosin in human vascular preparations. Archives Internationales de Pharmacodynamie et de Therapie 231: 81 (1978).

Kellaway, G.S.M.: Adverse drug reactions during treatment of hypertension. Drugs 11 (Suppl. 1): 91 (1976).

Kim, J.S.: A study of the use of prazosin in hypertensive patients in Korea. Clinical Science and Molecular Medicine 51: 45 (1976).

Kincaid-Smith, P.: Vasodilators in the treatment of hypertension. Medical Journal of Australia (Special Suppl) 1: 7 (1975).

Kincaid-Smith, Priscilla; Fang, P. and Laver, M.C.: A new look at the treatment of severe hypertension. Clinical Science and Molecular Medicine 45: 87S (1973).

Kincaid-Smith, Priscilla and Hua, A.: Beta-adrenergic blocking agents in renal failure. British Medical Journal 3: 520 (1974).

Kincaid-Smith, P.; Hua, A.S.P.; Myers, J.B.; Macdonald, I. and Fang, P.: Prazosin and hydrallazine in the treatment of hypertension. Paper presented at Symposium on Prazosin and Hypertension, Sydney, Melbourne and Auckland, Feb-Mar 1977.

Koshy, M.C.; Mickley, D.; Bourgoignie, J. and Blanfox, M.D.: Physiologic evaluation of a new antihypertensive agent: Prazosin HCl. Circulation 55: 533 (1977).

Kuokkanen, K. and Mattila, M.J.: Demonstration of an additive antihypertensive effect of prazosin and polythiazide in out-patients. Current Therapeutic Research 17: 431 (1975).

Lee, Y.W. and Seo, J.D.: A clinical study on antihypertensive effects of prazosin hydrochloride ('Minipress'). Korean Circulation Journal 5: 25 (1975).

Lowenthal, D.T.; Shirk, J.; Affrime, M.B.; Busby, P.; Kim, K.E.; Fernandes, M.; Martinez, E.W.; Onesti, G. and Swartz, C.D.: Pharmacokinetics and effectiveness of prazosin in patients with chronic renal failure. Clinical Pharmacology and Therapeutics 23: 119 (1978).

Lubbe, W.F.: Prazosin in the therapy of uncontrolled hypertension. South African Medical Journal 52: 913 (1977).

Lund-Johansen, P.: Hemodynamic changes at rest and during exercise in long term prazosin therapy of essential hypertension; in Cotton (Ed) Prazosin — Evaluation of a new antihypertensive agent (Excerpta Medica, Amsterdam, 1974).

Lund-Johansen, P.: Haemodynamic long-term effects of prazosin plus tolamolol in essential hypertension. British Journal of Clinical Pharmacology 4: 141 (1977).

Mabadeje, A.F.B.: An open trial of prazosin in the treatment of hypertension. Nigerian Medical Journal 8: 153 (1978).

Maher, P.H.: Clinical evaluation of prazosin in 20 private practice patients. Postgraduate Medicine (Suppl. Nov): 107 (1975).

Marshall, A.J.; Barritt, D.W.; Pocock, J. and Heaton, S.T.: Evaluation of beta-blockade, bendrofluazide, and prazosin in severe hypertension: Lancet 1: 271 (1977).

Martinez, E.W.; Fernandes, M.; Fiorentini, R.; Chandler, T.; Mazella, J.; Lowenthal, D.; Kim, K.E.; Swartz, C. and Onesti, G.: Effectiveness of the combination prazosin-propranolol-diuretic in refractory hypertension. Clinical Pharmacology and Therapeutics 23: 120 (1978).

Masoni, A.; Tommasi, A.M.; Baggioni, F. and Bagni, B.: Hemodynamic study in men of medium-term treatment with a new amino-quinazoline antihypertensive agent (prazosin); in Cotton (Ed) Prazosin — Evaluation of a new antihypertensive agent (Excerpta Medica, Amsterdam 1974).

Massingham, R. and Hayden, M.L.: A comparison of the effects of prazosin and hydrallazine on blood pressure, heart rate and plasma renin activity in conscious renal hypertensive dogs. European Journal of Pharmacology 30: 121 (1975).

Maxwell, M.H.: Effects of prazosin on renal function and fluid-electrolyte metabolism. Postgraduate Medicine (Suppl. Nov): 36 (1975).

Melkild, A.: Behandling av hypertensjon med prazosin ('Peripress') alene og i kombinasjon med beta-blokker: en apen undersokelse hos polikliniske pasienter. Current Medical Research and Opinion 4 (Suppl. 2): 69 (1977).

Moyer, R.R.: Experience with prazosin in a clinical setting. Postgraduate Medicine (Suppl. Nov): 101 (1975).

Mroczek, W.J. and Finnerty, F.A. Jr: Prazosin — a double blind evaluation; in Cotton (Ed) Prazosin — Evaluation of a new antihypertensive agent (Excerpta Medica, Amsterdam 1974).

Oates, H.F.; Graham, R.M.; Stoker, L.M. and Stokes, G.S.: Haemodynamic effects of prazosin. Archives internationales de pharmacodynamie et de therapie 224: 239 (1976).

Oates, H.F.; Graham, R.M. and Stokes, G.S.: Mechanism of the hypotensive action of prazosin. Archives Internationales de Pharmacodynamie et de Therapie 227: 41 (1977).

Oh, M.S.; Carroll, H.J.; Cruz, W.M.; Whang, E.S.M. and Lejano, R.F.: Treatment of hypertension with a combination of prazosin and polythiazide. Postgraduate Medicine (Suppl. Nov): 77 (1975).

Okun, R.: Dosage schedule routine for prazosin: two crossover trials comparing t.i.d. with q.i.d. administration and t.i.d. and b.i.d. administration; in Cotton (Ed) Prazosin — Evaluation of a new antihypertensive agent (Excerpta Medica, Amsterdam 1974).

Onesti, G.; Fernandes, M.A.; Kim, K.E. and Swartz, C.D.: Prazosin in the treatment of hypertension. Clinical Pharmacology and Therapeutics 15: 216 (1974).

Oviasu, V.O. and Idahosa, P.E.: Variability in effect of low doses of prazosin in hypertensive Nigerians. Current Therapeutic Research 20: 757 (1976).

Pape, J.; Saltvedt, E.; Westlie, L.; Shetelig, A. and Fauchald, P.: Prazosin i behandling av refroktaer hypertensjon. Current Medical Research and Opinion 4(Suppl. 2): 89 (1977).

Paul, R.R.; Sharma, P.L. and Wahi, P.L.: A phase II study of prazosin hydrochloride in hypertensive subjects. International Journal of Clinical Pharmacology 14: 271 (1974).

Pitkajarvi, T.; Kyostila, S.; Kontro, J. and Mattila, M.J.: Antihypertensive action of drug combination: polythiazide, prazosin and tolamolol. Current Therapeutic Research 21: 169 (1977).

Pitts, N.E.: The clinical evaluation of prazosin a new antihypertensive agent. Postgraduate Medicine (Suppl. Nov): 117 (1975).

Piza Lopez, A. and Gutierrez Fuster, E.: Study on the efficacy and tolerance of a new antihypertensive drug prazosin hydrochloride. Comparison with α-methyldopa. Investigacion Medica Internacional 3: 163 (1975).

Rab, S.M. and Farooqui, S.: Prazosin in the treatment of hypertension — a preliminary report. British Journal of Clinical Practice 29 (12): 337 (1975).

Raftos, J.: The difficult hypertensive. Drugs 11: 55 (1976).

Rand, M.J.; McCulloch, M.W. and Story, D.F.: Pre-junctional modulation of noradrenergic transmission by noradrenaline, dopamine and acetylcholine; in Davies and Reid (Eds) Central Action of Drugs in the Regulation of Blood Pressure (Pitman Medical, London 1975).

Rasmussen, K. and Jensen, H.A.: Prazosin in treatment of hypertension. British Medical Journal 4: 346 (1975).

Rasmussen, K. and Jensen, H.A.E.: A cross-over study between hydrallazine and prazosin. Clinical Science and Molecular Medicine 51: 612S (1976).

Rasmussen, K. and Jensen, H.A.: Prazosin og hydralazin: Ackvipotente antihypertensive doser i Kombinations-behandling med propranolol. Current Medical Research and Opinion 4(Suppl. 2): 77 (1977).

Rees, J. and Williams, H.: Adverse reactions to prazosin. British Medical Journal 3: 593 (1975).

Research Group, Japan.: Open studies with prazosin in the treatment of essential hypertension. Medical Journal of Australia 2(Suppl.): 38 (1977).

Reyes, A.L.: Prazosin; some clinical observations in ambulatory hypertensive patients. Philippine Journal of Cardiology 2: 30 (1974).

Roach, A.G.; Lefevre, F. and Cavero, I.: Effects of prazosin and phentolamine on cardiac presynaptic α-adrenoceptors in the cat, dog and rat. Clinical and Experimental Hypertension 1: 87 (1978).

Rosendorff, C.: Prazosin: severe side-effects are dose dependent. British Medical Journal 3: 508 (1976).

Rougier, M.; Lahon, H.F.J.; Clini, A.R.: Prazosin — a new antihypertensive agent. British Journal of Clinical Practice 28: 280 (1974).

Safar, M.E.; Weiss, Y.A.; London, G.L. and Milliez, P.L.: Short-term hemodynamic studies with prazosin; in Cotton (Ed) Prazosin — Evaluation of a new antihypertensive agent (Excerpta Medica, Amsterdam 1974).

Salim, S.S.; Mtui, E.P.J. and Makene, W.J.: An open evaluation of the efficacy and toleration of prazosin in patients with hypertension. East African Medical Journal 54: 429 (1977).

Schnaper, H.W. and Oberman, A.: Double-blind studies of the clinical effectiveness of prazosin. Postgraduate Medicine (Suppl. Nov): 81 (1975).

Schirger, A. and Sheps, S.G.: Prazosin — a new antihypertensive agent. A double-blind crossover study in the treatment of hypertension. Journal of the American Medical Association 237: 989 (1977).

Scivoletto, R.; Toledo, A.J.O.; Gomes da Silva, A.C. and Nigro, D.: Mechanism of the hypotensive effect of prazosin. Archives internationales de pharmacodynamie et de therapie 223: 333 (1976).

Seedat, Y.K.: Treatment of hypertension with the aid of beta-adrenergic blocking drugs. South African Medical Journal 48: 846 (1975).

Seedat, Y.K.: Bhoola, R. and Rampono, J.G.: Prazosin in treatment of hypertension. British Medical Journal 3: 305 (1975b).

Seedat, Y.K.; North-Coombes, D. and Rampono, J.G.: Prazosin in the treatment of hypertension. South African Medical Journal Mediese Tydskrif 49: 1741 (1975a).

Seedat, Y.K.; Seedat, M.A. and Bhoola, R.: Prazosin alone and combined with a thiazide diuretic in the treatment of hypertension. South African Medical Journal 51: 461 (1977).

Simpson, F.O.: Some aspects of the pharmacology of prazosin and their clinical implications. Medical Journal of Australia 2 (Suppl.): 7 (1977).

Simpson, F.O.; Bolli, P. and Wood, J.: Use of prazosin at the Dunedin hypertensive clinic. Controlled and open studies and pharmacokinetic observations. Medical Journal of Australia 2 (Suppl.): 17 (1977).

Smith, I.S.; Fernandes, M.; Kim, K.E.; Swartz, C. and Onesti, G.: A three-phase clinical evaluation of prazosin. Postgraduate Medicine (Suppl. Nov): 53 (1975).

Steele, J.M. and Lowenstein, J.: Absence of renin stimulation of tachycardia during antihypertensive therapy with prazosin. Presented at the 4th meetings of the International Society of Hypertension, Sydney (February, 1976).

Stokes, G.S.; Gain, J.M.; Mahony, J.F.; Stewart, J.H. and Raftos, J.: Long-term use of prazosin in combination or alone for treating hypertension. Medical Journal of Australia 2 (Suppl.): 13 (1977a).

Stokes, G.S.; Graham, R.M.; Gain, J.M. and Davis, P.R.: Influence of dosage and dietary sodium on the first-dose effects of prazosin. British Medical Journal 1: 1507 (1977).

Stokes, G.S. and Oates, H.F.: Comparative and interaction studies with peripherally-acting hypotensive agents. Special supplement to the Medical Journal of Australia 2: 9 (1977b).

Stokes, G.S. and Weber, M.A.: Prazosin: preliminary report and comparative studies with other antihypertensive agents. British Medical Journal 2: 298 (1974).

Taylor, J.A.; Twomey, T.M. and Schach von Wittenau, M.: The metabolic fate of prazosin. Xenobiotica. In press (1976).

Thulin, J.A.; Saetre, H.; Vikesdahl, O.; Warmenius, S.; Persson, G. and Schersten, B.: Multicenter study of the antihypertensive effects of prazosin hydrochloride (prazosin) on mild and moderate hypertension; in Cotton (Ed) Prazosin — Evaluation of a new antihypertensive agent (Excerpta Medica, Amsterdam 1974).

Turner, A.S.: Prescribing prazosin. New Zealand Medical Journal 84: 31 (1976a).

Turner, A.S.: Prazosin in hypertension. British Medical Journal 2: 1257 (1976b).

Turner, A.S.; Watson, O.F. and Brocklehurst, J.E.: Prazosin in hypertension. Clinical studies with special reference to initiation of therapy. Medical Journal of Australia 2 (Suppl.): 33 (1977).

Turner, A.S.; Watson, O. and Peel, J.S.: Clinical experience with prazosin hydrochloride in arterial hypertension. New Zealand Medical Journal 81: 240 (1975).

Venables, T.L. and Duff, R.S.: A comparative trial of prazosin and methyldopa; in Cotton (Ed) Prazosin — Evaluation of a new antihypertensive agent (Excerpta Medica, Amsterdam 1974).

Verbesselt, R.; Mullie, A.; Tjandramaga, T.B.; De Schepper, P.J. and Dessain, P.: The effect of food intake on the plasma kinetics and toleration of prazosin. Acta Therapeutica 2: 27 (1976).

Verhiest, W.; Croonenberghs, J.; Devos, P.; Fagard, R. and Amery, A.: Double-blind cross-over study comparing prazosin and methyldopa in the treatment of mild hypertension. Acta Cardiologica 29: 217 (1974).

Vyrens, R. and Adriaensen, H.: Double-blind crossover comparative study with low doses of prazosin and α-methyldopa; in Cotton (Ed) Prazosin — Evaluation of a new antihypertensive agent (Excerpta Medica, Amsterdam 1974).

Wood, A.J.: Pharmacokinetics of prazosin in man. Presented to the Annual Meeting of the Australasian Society of Clinical and Experimental Pharmacologists, December 1974; see also Clinical and Experimental Pharmacology and Physiology 2: 446 (1975).

Wood, A.J.; Bolli, B. and Simpson, F.O.: Prazosin in normal subjects: plasma levels, blood pressure and heart rate. British Journal of Clinical Pharmacology 1: 199 (1976).

Wood, A.J. and Lee, D.R.: Effects of prazosin on sodium and body fluids in genetically hypertensive rats. Proceedings of the University of Otago Medical School 52: 12 (1974).

Wood, A.J.; Phelan, E.L. and Simpson, F.O.: Cardiovascular effects of prazosin in normotensive and genetically hypertensive rats. Clinical and Experimental Pharmacology and Physiology 2: 297 (1975).

Zapala, H.H. and Bengolea, A.M.: Clinical experience with prazosin in essential blood hypertension therapy (translation). Prensa Medica Argentina 60: 1227 (1973).

Subject Index